T0198267

Facial Deformities in Children
Thirteen Life-Changing Operations

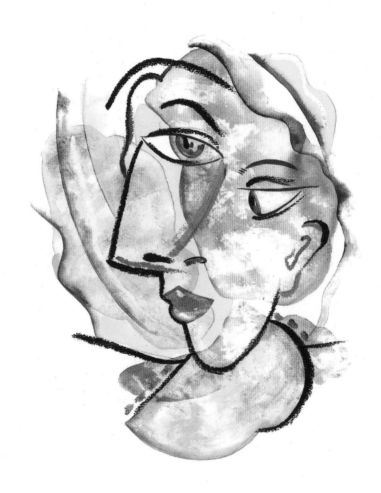

Facial Deformities in Children
Thirteen Life-Changing Operations

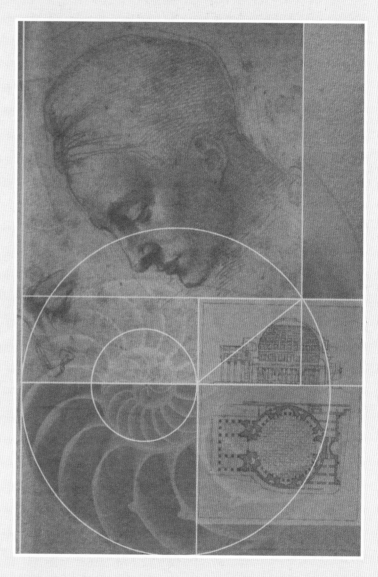

JEFFREY C. POSNICK,
DMD, MD, FRCS(C), FACS

Professor Emeritus, Plastic and Reconstructive
  Surgery and Pediatrics
Georgetown University School of Medicine
Washington, DC

Professor of Orthodontics
University of Maryland, Baltimore College of
  Dental Surgery
Baltimore, Maryland

Professor of Oral and Maxillofacial Surgery
Howard University College of Dentistry
Washington, DC

Adjunct Professor of Plastic and Reconstructive
  Surgery
Johns Hopkins School of Medicine,
Baltimore, Maryland

Posnick MD Consulting, LLC
Potomac, Maryland

ELSEVIER

Elsevier
3251 Riverport Lane
St. Louis, Missouri 63043

FACIAL DEFORMITIES IN CHILDREN: THIRTEEN LIFE-CHANGING OPERATIONS   ISBN: 978-0-323-93239-4
Copyright © 2024 by Jeffrey C. Posnick. Published by Elsevier Inc.

Notice

Practitioners and researchers must always rely on their own experience and knowledge in evaluating and using any information, methods, compounds or experiments described herein. Because of rapid advances in the medical sciences, in particular, independent verification of diagnoses and drug dosages should be made. To the fullest extent of the law, no responsibility is assumed by Elsevier, authors, editors or contributors for any injury and/or damage to persons or property as a matter of products liability, negligence or otherwise, or from any use or operation of any methods, products, instructions, or ideas contained in the material herein.

Unless otherwise indicated, medical illustrations throughout the work © by Elsevier Inc.

Content Strategist: Lauren Boyle
Content Development Specialist: Grace Onderlinde
Project Manager: Anne Collett
Design Direction: Brian Salisbury

Printed in India

Last digit is the print number: 9 8 7 6 5 4 3 2 1

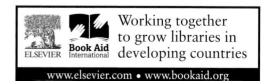

Reviews

The spectrum of careers in medicine is rarely covered adequately in pre-residency training. Sub-specialty surgical careers are the most vulnerable to this exclusion. Graduates often need to decide what path to take too early in their training, without ever understanding all the exciting choices open to them. Dr. Posnick's text *13 Life-Changing Operations* is an invaluable resource for any student wishing to explore the rewards and challenges of a career in craniofacial reconstructive surgery. Using succinct clinical summaries followed by thoughtful preoperative, intraoperative, and postoperative images, Posnick walks the reader through a series of complex reconstructive surgeries that display the full spectrum of his specialty. Novel to surgical texts, *13 Life-Changing Operations* also includes an insight into the impact these procedures have had on people's lives, through letters and images sent to Dr. Posnick from grateful families. It provides an insight into a critical privilege that craniofacial surgeons enjoy in being able to follow patients from birth to maturity and connect with their patients in a profound way. Finally, resting on decades of experience, Posnick shares his perspectives on what it means to be a surgeon, and how to excel in the field. As a fellow surgeon in his third decade of craniofacial surgery I thoroughly enjoyed reading this new book by Jeffrey Posnick and am glad it is now available to the new generation of trainees exploring this exciting and rewarding field.

Richard A. Hopper, MD
Marlys C. Larson Chair of Craniofacial Surgery
Professor, University of Washington
Seattle, WA, United States

In this text, Dr. Posnick focuses on the most transformative craniofacial surgeries for children. In each of 13 operations described, he covers the biology of the condition and history of the procedure, as well as the technical aspects of the operation. It is succinct and very clearly illustrated with abundant diagrams and clinical photos showing results that are breathtaking. Perhaps most significantly, it is populated with letters from grateful children and parents, some 10–20 years postoperatively, testifying to the profound impact that the surgery had on their lives and how it shaped their futures for the better. Dr. Posnick shows that he is nothing short of a grand master of his profession, but his focus on the effect these surgeries have on the child's sense of self is sure to inspire generations of students to follow in his footsteps.

Larry H. Hollier Jr, MD
Surgeon-in-Chief and Chair of Surgery
Texas Children's Hospital
Houston, TX, United States

DEDICATION

This book is in honor of parents who love, siblings who support, and surgeons who reconstruct children born with facial deformity.

Parents provide a safe, consistent, and caring home environment, enabling their child to explore the world.

Siblings provide unconditional friendship and support, encouraging their brother or sister to interact with others.

Pioneer surgeons inspire future generations of physicians to go further.

Contents

Foreword

PAUL N. MANSON

This is a unique book, written by a world-class craniofacial and orthognathic surgeon after his retirement. He has previously authored what, in my opinion, is the best text on the subject, *Orthognathic Surgery: Principles and Practice*, which has recently published its second edition (Elsevier, 2022) and teaches the number 1 Orthognathic Surgery course in the world for the AO Foundation. The purpose of this present book is to inform and guide parents of children with congenital, neoplastic, and accidental facial deformities, permitting understanding from the standpoint of someone who has treated thousands of children, and guided their parents to better understanding of the deformities, their treatment, and to management of the procedural, logistical, and emotional issues common to the patients and the families. I know this information is something that Dr. Posnick has felt strongly about, which he now communicates from the perspective of someone who gives (not being in active practice) unconflicted advice and perspective from the experience of his years in service.

Unique in this book are the initial and final chapters, which detail sage advice for parents: My Story (about Posnick himself); About Surgery and Surgeons; About Surgical Preparation; and Perspectives on Facial Aesthetics. Later, at the end of the book are chapters on Future Directions in the field of facial reconstruction; and the author's Final Thoughts. The chapter on Future Directions describes the exciting future, with better imaging, biomaterials, analytic and predictive techniques, virtual surgical planning, prosthetic advance, molecular biology, operating rooms of the future, pharmaceuticals, health care of the future, and artificial intelligence. The 13 chapters that form the body of the book each deal with various aspects of the more common diagnoses, to include history, diagnostic criteria, treatment options, spectrum of findings, possible operations and their goals, prognosis, with pictures of before and after, technique illustrations, descriptions of possibilities and choices, and principles of treatment selection, and letters revealing patient experiences.

When I was a resident in the 1970s I can recall my chief asking me, when he received a call about a child with a particularly wide and challenging cleft of the lip and palate, if I wanted to go with him to view an urgent consultation from another hospital's newborn care unit. They were desperate to get advice and hope, and to receive information by consultation which would calm the family and the pediatricians and nurses caring for the child. They were experiencing feeding difficulties for the child, as well as being perplexed about a condition they feared was not surgically treatable. There, the professor approached the problem with reassurance, and in a calm and assured conversation, stressed that the problem "just needs to be fixed" by someone (him) with skill and special training. His firm and certain explanation calmed all parties, and he then proceeded to inform the nurses how to feed the child to get the growth and nourishment to prepare the child for surgery several months later, when the stresses of newborn status and birth were past.

Today, these diagnoses are usually made in this country before birth, and counseling in a predictive and relaxed fashion can be accomplished prenatally. This book contains 13 chapters, selected by the author as frequent and at first almost overwhelming conditions, which are definitively managed by surgery with the fear and apprehension greatly improved and resolved by information, statistics, and experience. That information, which comes from an extremely experienced practitioner, who has spent his life counseling families and patients, and treating these conditions, is here for all to benefit from. I know this book is something Dr. Posnick has been thinking about for years, and strongly believes in.

Dr. Posnick's career, summarized in the book's introductory materials, is an educational paradigm I came to favor after training many, many residents. Posnick and I each came to this format independently, he for himself, and me for very talented and dedicated residents who wished to be at the top of their profession. We are both strong believers in these educational principles. Only someone so thoroughly and accurately trained could produce a textbook such as his *Orthognathic Surgery* as a single author (most books are multi-authored). Indeed, the educational process described produces some of the world's most talented and capable craniofacial and orthognathic surgeons, and requires the rather extreme commitment of a 15–20-year period of education and training. The training begins with medical and dental schools. Then, basic training in the surgical disciplines of plastic and reconstructive surgery and oral and maxillofacial surgery is followed by fellowships in craniofacial surgery, orthognathic surgery, then finished with aesthetic and head and neck surgery experience. Frequently, the best programs require a year of research and the clinical requirements as "payback" for the individuals running those programs. This broad multidisciplinary training produces single individuals cable of understanding and practicing multiple disciplines for the most challenging conditions. The training produces surgeons whose comprehensive knowledge base allows complete treatment led by single talented individuals, avoiding the disorganization of treatment plans generated by groups of single-specialty surgeon specialists. Their multidisciplinary teams are led with experience and direction not equaled by individual specialty practitioners, but the latter are still part of a team and directed with wise integration from leadership.

In this present book, advice, thoughts, and "pearls" are provided so that parents and families may follow the recommendations to produce a roadmap to the best and most thorough resolution possible. This book provides valuable pathways and advice for a group of 13 conditions usually not emphasized or not having the benefit of common knowledge information because of their less common incidence.

My grateful thanks go to Dr. Posnick and the publishers for recognizing and for producing materials which are pertinent and highly informative. They will certainly provide much comfort and information for those who experience these conditions in their families.

Paul N. Manson, MD
Distinguished Service Professor
Johns Hopkins University School of Medicine
Professor, University of Maryland Shock Trauma Unit,
and the Department of Surgery
University of Maryland School of Medicine
Baltimore, MA, United States

Foreword

TIMOTHY A. TURVEY

Dr. Posnick has done it again! After authoring two comprehensive landmark textbooks on orthognathic and craniofacial surgery, directed to professionals, this prolific author has completed a wonderful treatise directed at students and others, including non-professionals, who may have an interest in pursuing surgery as a career to help the facially disfigured. Additionally, Posnick directs the work towards those who would be potential contributors to improving access to care issues for patients with facial deformities.

After 16 years of post-collegiate training, Dr. Posnick entered the craniofacial surgical arena at the Hospital for Sick Children in Toronto, before relocating to Washington, DC. In Washington, he established a private practice dedicated to facial reconstructive surgery. Eighteen months after retiring from this practice and with more than 30 years of surgical experience, Dr. Posnick has produced this wonderful treatise based on his vast experience and expertise.

The monograph highlights 13 life-changing operations with photos and illustrations describing the procedures, which range from unusual transcranial skull remodeling and orbital hypertelorism correction, to the mundane cosmetic rhinoplasty. The point is that each of these procedures is capable of making a positive impact on a patient's quality of life. The emphasis is not so much on the physical change associated with these operations, although very impressive, but more on the patients' appreciation of the changes and improvement in self-confidence, self-concept, and self-image that they have experienced. The reader cannot help being overcome by the gratification that this surgeon's career must have brought to him in treating so many. As a parent of a child who underwent this type of surgery, Dr. Posnick has also experienced the anguish involved with the decision to accept this surgery for one of his own and has witnessed the remarkable changes both physically and psychosocially.

The book does not have the same detail that would be in a text directed to a professional audience. It is well illustrated, and the photographic documentation tells the story.

Just as Dr. Joseph Murray and Dr. Paul Tessier influenced Dr. Posnick's decision to pursue this surgical pathway, this monograph will have a similar influence on the career of the next generation of surgeons dedicating their practices to the facially disfigured. It is a must read for anyone thinking about a very gratifying surgical career.

Timothy A. Turvey DDS, FACS
*Professor, Department of Craniofacial
and Surgical Services
University of North Carolina
Chapel Hill, NC, United States*

Introduction and My Story

JEFFREY C. POSNICK, DMD, MD

The purpose of this monograph is to share knowledge about the spectrum of facial deformities in children. They occur in everyday life, regardless of the individual's cultural background or economic status. Pioneer physicians have described and detailed these conditions over many decades. As innovative surgeons strive to make improvements for affected children and young adults, more work needs to be done!

This is about the inescapable cruelty of facial deformity in children. The benefits of reconstructive surgery and the challenges that remain as told from the perspective of my life's work, after decades as a pediatric facial surgeon, educator, clinical researcher in the field, and as a father whose son required reconstructive jaw surgery.

My hope is that after reading and considering this text, some who have not yet committed to a profession may be inspired to make this their life's work. Others may decide to support needed research, provide funding for clinical care, advocate at a state or federal level, or just be more empathetic to those who live with these special challenges.

My story begins with a father raised by first-generation immigrants from eastern Europe. He was the first in his family to not only complete high school but to attend college. He married his high school sweetheart, graduated from dental school, served as an officer in the US Navy during World War II and, once back in civilian life, opened a dental practice in his hometown of Minneapolis, Minnesota. My mother was a homemaker and, together, they raised four boys. Just as my father, the four of us also attended public schools, including college, and then graduated from dental school. My path diverged from theirs when I accepted a position at Harvard School of Dental Medicine. At that time, life in the northeast at an Ivy League graduate school was a very different cultural experience from that in the midwest at a public university. Once in Boston, I felt a surge of inadequacy and intimidation in an environment that exuded sophistication and brilliance. My new contemporaries were graduates from Harvard, Yale, and Princeton who seemed so much smarter than me. They included Rhodes Scholars, newly minted PhDs in biochemistry, and all seemed to have gone to prestigious prep schools. Only later would I appreciate that my midwestern upbringing and public schooling stood me well. Early in my dental education I attended an evening seminar offered by Dr. Joseph Murray, the newly appointed Professor and Chief of Pediatric Plastic Surgery at Boston Children's Hospital and Harvard Medical School. Murray is best known for having completed the first successful human kidney transplant (December 23, 1954), for which he later received the Nobel Prize (1990). By the early 1970s he became devoted to the new field of reconstructive surgery, specifically for the correction of facial deformities in children. His lecture to our group of Harvard dental students (class of 1977) was about facial deformities in children and what a surgeon, at that time, could accomplish. The special challenges that the children and their families faced were disturbing to us, but the pioneer reconstructive surgeries described were inspiring! I gradually got to know Dr. Murray while attending hospital teaching rounds and was then introduced to his young faculty: Lenny Kaban (oral and maxillofacial surgeon) and John Mullikan (plastic surgeon). Lenny agreed to advise me through dental school and then became a lifelong mentor. Dr. Paul Tessier (pioneer craniofacial surgeon in Paris, France), during that time, scheduled regular visits to Boston Children's Hospital to work with the team evaluating patients and then carrying out complex craniofacial surgery. Murray and Tessier recognized blind spots in their own education and understood the unique advantages of analyzing facial deformities in children and then executed craniofacial surgery both from the perspective of dentistry (Oral and Maxillofacial Surgery) and medicine (Plastic Surgery). As mentors, they encouraged me to train in both fields and I did.

After graduating dental school, I gained advanced standing at Vanderbilt Medical School. I then trained in Oral and Maxillofacial Surgery, completed a surgical internship at Vanderbilt and a second and third year of General Surgery at Massachusetts General Hospital. Next was a Pediatric Craniofacial Surgery Fellowship at the Children's Hospital of Philadelphia and, as Drs. Murray and Tessier suggested, a full residency in Plastic Surgery. After completing training, I accepted a position at The Hospital for Sick Children and the University of Toronto as head of the Pediatric Craniofacial Surgery Program.

My 16 years of undergraduate and graduate education and residency training may be viewed by some as a prolonged and tortuous road, but I considered it a privilege, appreciating the opportunity to gain medical knowledge and learn surgical skills. It was all immensely helpful in the years to come when caring for children born with or having acquired a facial deformity.

During my dental school years, I observed the Boston surgical team month after month, as they worked through complex facial reconstructions in children, agonizing over the outcomes and then modifying techniques for the next patient. I learned to incorporate their habit of critical thinking with a commitment to the scientific method but always remembering that the goal had to be a better life for the individual child under my care. This still sums up my way of thinking. Gaining insight from Paul Tessier was another great advantage. I initially observed his work with the Boston Children's team, then I assisted Tessier while a Plastic Surgery resident and then visited him later in Paris. Over the years he taught me the necessity of hard work, the importance of being organized in the operating room, the need for confidence, determination, and the value of individualistic thinking.

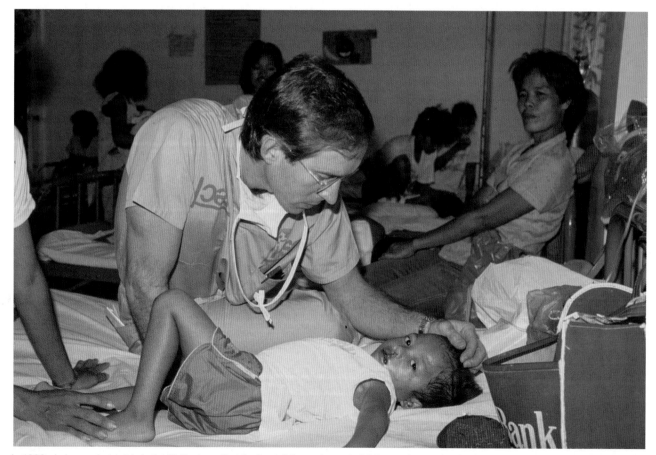

• In 1986, during a mission trip in the Philippines. Repair of a cleft lip maybe a straightforward operation for the surgeon but it is a life-changing event for the child.

About Surgery and Surgeons

JEFFREY C. POSNICK, DMD, MD

Surgery joins a unique family of professions that help others: firefighters run into burning buildings, police officers charge towards danger, and surgeons use their hands to find and remove disease and correct deformities. A surgeon takes action as an individual, not as a committee or institution. A surgeon is never anonymous. Surgeons make the critical decisions alone, utilizing their own brains and hands to accomplish objectives. Once an operation begins, the tasks cannot be delegated, postponed, or debated.

Emergency surgery, such as managing a gunshot wound to the chest, a ruptured heart valve, or an infected appendix, typically requires the rapid transfer of the patient to the operating room, often with limited time to confirm the diagnosis or to contemplate all treatment options. From a surgeon's perspective, reducing a fracture, managing an infection, or cleaning and repairing a wound can be satisfying work, but going a step further and performing elective surgery is another thing entirely. The term elective surgery implies that there is time to fully clarify the diagnosis and to consider the spectrum of options before proceeding. Unless there is uncontrolled hemorrhage, a rapidly progressing infection, or imminent airway compromise, all head and neck procedures are considered elective.

For non-emergency "elective" surgery, there are always options about what to do and when to do it. Each choice has its own set of risks and theoretical advantages. When the operating surgeon discusses the risks and potential benefits of each option with the patient/family, the conversation comes from a perspective of the surgeon's own experiences. It would be naive to think that the surgeon's unique past experiences do not heavily influence their recommended option. When the surgeon recommends a specific operation, there may be safer alternatives that offer less potential upside. Ideally, the choice should always fit the patient's needs and not the surgeon's personal skill set. The decision is even more difficult when it is for a child, who cannot directly offer informed consent.

For the surgeon, a healthy degree of confidence is always beneficial to gain the trust of the patient/family and to have the fortitude to proceed. Surgical confidence is achieved through a long process of in-depth education, rigorous training, and extensive experience. An experienced and confident surgeon is more likely to make an accurate diagnosis, choose the appropriate course of action, and safely execute the operation. As each operation has a learning curve and each patient's conditions are unique, surgeons are forced to make decisions with levels of uncertainty and to accept the responsibility that follows.

Surgeons are by necessity lifelong learners. The daily exposure to new ideas and the incorporation of advanced knowledge and innovative techniques into clinical practice is invigorating. However, surgeons can get in the habit of doing things in a certain way "because it works." Exceptional surgeons do not continue using the same procedure without a reason that can be defended. Having a curious mind to ask the right questions, using imagination to connect ideas and observations, and being persistent and tenacious is part of the process. Engaged surgeons always seek better ways to solve old problems. Working at a teaching hospital and interacting with surgeons-in-training is a great advantage. Students tend to question medical dogma providing opportunities to find new solutions to old problems. Often I have found that even the best ideas require rethinking and time to mature.

The process of articulating a new idea on paper and incorporating it into the bigger picture helps to clarify knowledge on the subject.

The phrase "embrace change" has become a popular notion in our culture. For a surgeon to abandon a technique that works reasonably well, there should be proof of the concept that the new way is better. For example, we were told that "tissue expanders" would revolutionize all forms of reconstructive surgery. In reality, they have found a useful but limited role. A surgeon knows too well that the consequences of a bad idea can cause irreversible harm to their patient. Being curious, asking the right questions, making clinical observations but always clarifying the facts through the scientific method should guide the process.

Well-grounded surgeons learn to accept what is out of their control and forgive themselves for occasional errors as long as they have thoughtfully done their best. A good rule of thumb is to never do anything that would shame your mentor. Despite best efforts, all active clinical surgeons will experience complications in their patients. The important aspect is to learn from each of these challenges and never repeat the same mistake.

It is a human quality to want to be of help to others. What greater gift than to acquire the knowledge of medicine and the skills of surgery and then to use those talents to help others in need! The joys of being a surgeon are immense and include:

- being a detective, gathering information in support of making the correct diagnosis
- preparing for and completing a well-planned and successfully executed operation
- being of help to others and, when you least expect it, receiving gratitude from a patient and family
- constantly being exposed to new ideas and technologies
- learning from and working with respected colleagues
- teaching others what you have learned
- and hopefully advancing science.

You do not have to be the surgeon on the team to provide a helping hand to the child in need. In the operating room, the immediate team is extensive and includes: the surgeon and their assistants; the anesthesiologist and their assistants; the scrub nurse and circulating nurse; medical instruments (i.e., products and sterilization, packaging, and distribution personnel); medical device equipment (products and personnel support); and the front desk communication and administration support (i.e., technology and personnel). Without strong spokes of the wheel the wagon will not reach its destination. This is true for the entire hospital team. From the moment the child and their parents arrive, the system moves into action. The admission, preoperative testing, and preoperative holding teams prior to surgery are essential to ensure safe surgery. After surgery, the recovery room, intensive care unit, hospital ward, and discharge teams guide the child to a soft landing. Each team is composed of doctors, nurses, and therapists, and all must be supported by logistical personnel (i.e., cleaning, transportation, purchasing, security, safety, medical records, technology support, administration).

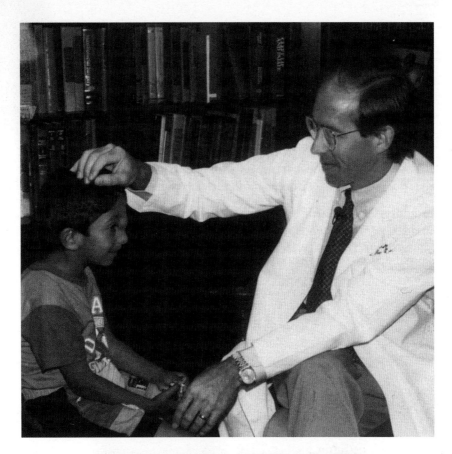

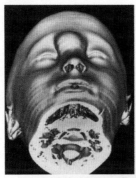 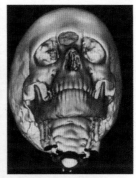

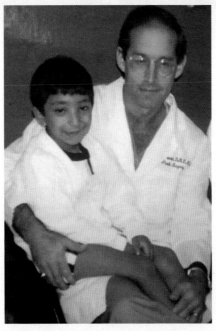

• A 7-year-old child from Romania, sent to me by the Save the Children charity in 1994. The encephalocele malformation was repaired and the skull defect reconstructed. He then returned home to a new life filled with hope.

About Surgical Preparation

JEFFREY C. POSNICK, DMD, MD

Most surgical challenges are won or lost before they start. The advantage goes to those that realize the potential difficulties in advance and then choose the terrain on which the battle is fought.

Experienced surgeons ask themselves in advance what difficulties might occur. Being knowledgeable, disciplined, and meticulous means that when a surgical challenge arises you are able to think it through. When a problem emerges, you will respond favorably.

An operation will generally go well if the indications are clear, and the procedure is thoroughly planned. A methodical surgeon will have considered the details in advance and then prepared the team. In surgery, having an effective strategy is everything. Mastering technical skills of the procedure is the easy part. Good judgment is the difficult part, knowing what to do and when to do it.

A useful rule of thumb is to practice surgery with reverence for the past, relevance for the present, and leadership towards the future.

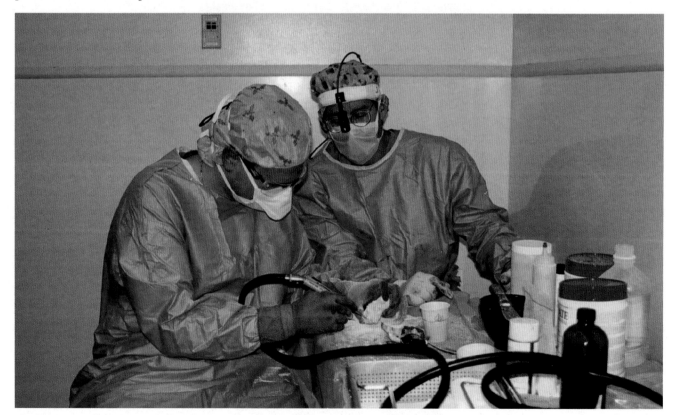

• During a surgical procedure in 1998. My Fellow (Ramon Ruiz) and I are preparing materials in the operating room on the back table for a child's skull reconstruction.

Perspectives on Facial Aesthetics

JEFFREY C. POSNICK, DMD, MD

Optimal facial proportions and mirror image symmetry attract positive emotional interest and move us to engage the person behind the face.
Facial disproportion and asymmetry are at best emotionally distancing and tend to discourage us towards social engagement.

We use the word proportion or balance to describe the comparative relationship between different parts or traits in an attempt to understand harmonious relationships between these parts and the whole. A definition of beauty can be found in Webster's unabridged dictionary as "the quality which makes an object seem pleasing or satisfying in a certain way." Optimal proportions are found in all forms of art, and throughout the centuries. Objects of classic beauty and the most attractive forms in nature consistently reveal the "Golden Ratio." From Pythagoras, Euclid, Da Vinci, and more recently Le Corbusier, we have learned that the proportions of the parts to the whole affect the observer's impression of beauty and attractiveness. Why? Neurobiologists tell us that the limbic structures of the central nervous system are primal components that regulate our emotional perceptions of visual stimuli. When one human views another at conversational distance, unless they sense a certain degree of harmony and mirror image symmetry in the face, the limbic component of their brain finds it disquieting and uncomfortable. The instinct is to either disengage or in some other way distance or shut out the image centered in their visual field. This is a primal instinct that is difficult to overcome. A person can learn to rise above this instinct, but it takes concentrated mental effort and consistent emotional restraint. Studies also confirm the detrimental effects on the individual who must sustain constant negative input and unremitting social stigma from their visible facial deformity. For these reasons, it is not enough for a craniofacial or maxillofacial surgeon to improve the affected individual's "function" (i.e., cognitive, vision, hearing, speech, chewing, swallowing, breathing) but meticulous attention should also be directed to the child's facial aesthetics which affects their body image and self-esteem.

I have come to appreciate that all facial disfigurements, even relatively minor deformities, have the potential to cause unnecessary anguish (see Chapter 13). The children highlighted in this monograph certainly fall into this category and the operations described offer them a way out. The next generation of surgeons will continue to innovate, improve the safety of the surgery, and provide broader access to these life-changing reconstructive procedures.

Letter About a Past Patient

Dear Dr. Posnick,

It is our sincere pleasure to write to you today thanking you for your role in caring for a former patient, Samuel Thames. You may recall Samuel's story. He was born with multiple health conditions which his birth family was not able to care for. He was adopted as a newborn by Reverend Thames. As an infant you led the team that provided exceptional care requiring multiple surgeries. Today, Samuel is a healthy and happy adult who has excelled in all of his efforts and lives an independent and wholesome life. He teaches at Drake University and, with a compassion for the disadvantaged, he acts as a mentor

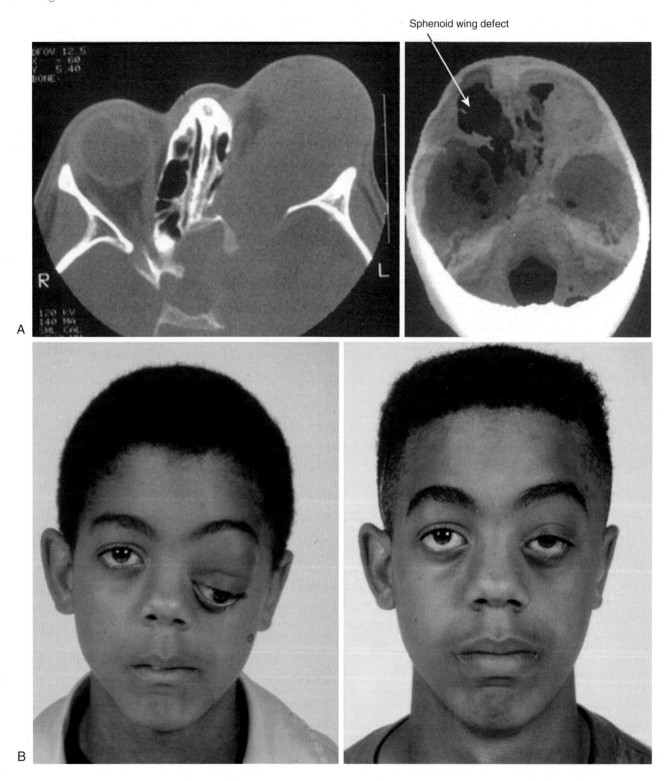

A child with neurofibromatosis involving the left cranio-orbital region. Aplasia of the sphenoid wing and the gradual growth of plexiform neurofibroma occurred, which extended from the cavernous sinus through the widened superior orbital fissure, through the cone of the eye, and into the upper eyelid. This resulted in distortion and proptosis of the left eye. The vision remained intact. The patient underwent transcranial reconstruction of the cranio-orbito-zygomatic skeleton, including the debulking of the soft-tissue tumor and upper eyelid reconstruction. **A,** CT scan views indicating the defect of the sphenoid wing and the extent of neurofibromatosis. **B,** Frontal facial views before and several years after surgery with good vision. (From Posnick JC, Selected complex malformations. Orthognathic Surgery: Principles and Practice, 2nd ed. [JC Posnick, ed., B. Kinard, assoc. ed.]. Saint Louis: Elsevier. Chapter 31, Figure 31-6, pp.1530-1531; 2022.)

1

Reconstruction of Isolated Craniosynostosis

JEFFREY C. POSNICK, DMD, MD

The flat bones of the cranial vault begin to develop during embryologic life. This process continues after birth, in synchrony, to match the shape and volume needs of the expanding, underlying brain. The separate bones of the skull accommodate the rapid brain growth that occurs in infancy through unique connections to one another, called "sutures". The connecting sutures stretch when under expansion pressure from the growing brain and in so doing, the cranial vault takes on a characteristic expected "normal" shape.

Craniosynostosis is the condition of premature fusion of a cranial suture(s) that occurs between one or more of the bones of the skull before the brain completes its rapid phase of growth during the first 18 months of life. When a cranial vault suture fuses prematurely during fetal development, a distinctive and characteristic abnormal shape to the head will be present at birth. The characteristic dysmorphology (abnormal shape) is dependent on the specific suture line closure and may result in, for example: trigonocephaly (i.e., metopic suture synostosis); anterior plagiocephaly (i.e., coronal suture synostosis); or scaphocephaly (i.e., sagittal suture synostosis) (see Figs. 1.1–1.3).

The pioneer human pathologist Rudolf Virchow of Würzberg, Germany was the first to take an interest in this malformation. In the 1850s, postmortem studies of craniosynostosis skulls were directly correlated to the observed abnormal head shapes. By doing so, Virchow was able to explain a relationship between the premature suture(s) fusion, the observed skull dysmorphology, and the resulting brain compression.[1]

We now know that if a cranial vault with premature suture synostosis is not surgically expanded in infancy, a degree of brain compression with negative effects on the child's cognitive ability can be expected.[2,3] For this reason, surgical release of the child's fused suture(s) to expand the intracranial volume and to simultaneously reconstruct the abnormal head shape should be undertaken. When the surgery is optimally timed and the region of dysmorphology is precisely reconstructed a single procedure is all that should be required (see Figs. 1.1–1.3).[4]

Advances in the fields of molecular biology and genetics, as well as the use of animal models have been of great importance in expanding our knowledge of craniosynostosis. Despite these advances, the preferred age (between 6 and 18 months) during childhood for the surgical expansion of the skull remains under study. The optimal extent of cranial vault and upper orbital reconstruction (i.e., the bones that house the brain and eyes) for the affected child also continues to be debated.[5,6] The answers to these questions and further refinements for the safety of craniosynostosis surgery remains for the future.[7,8]

Letter from a Past Patient

Dear Dr. Posnick,

I wanted you to know how very grateful I am for the most wonderful job you did on my head. I am now turning 11 years of age. My parents say that I was only 10 months old when you performed the skull surgery. I have really grown a lot since then. I love the outdoors - camping and fishing are the best. I am active in swimming and soccer. I will be going into the 5th grade in September. My mom tells me every day what a beautiful boy I am and that someday I should thank you for what you have done for me. Thank you so much for making me look and feel the way I do.

Yours truly,
Ben Johnson

📄

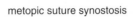

metopic suture synostosis

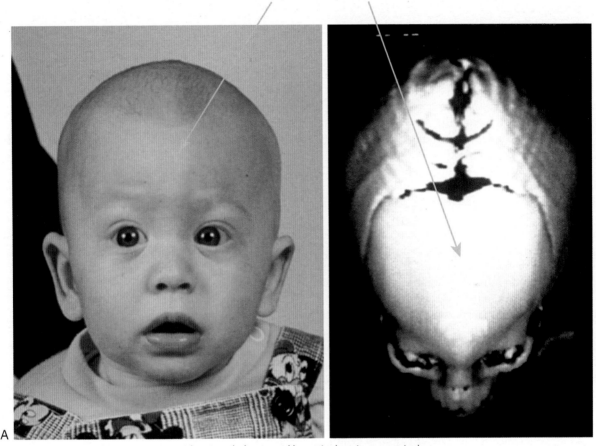

trigonocephaly: caused by metopic suture synostosis

• **Figure 1.1** A child born with metopic synostosis resulting in trigonocephaly. He underwent anterior cranial vault and three-quarter orbital osteotomies with reshaping at 10 months of age. **A**, Facial and computed tomography (CT) scan views prior to surgery.

Continued

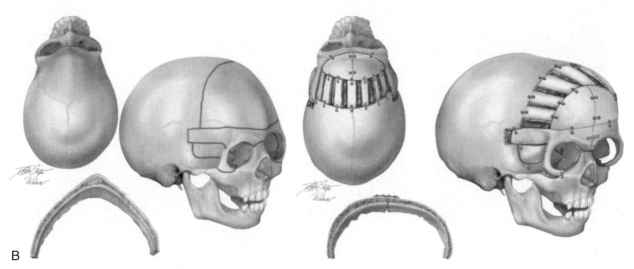

B   illustrations before & after reconstruction of the cranial vault & upper orbits

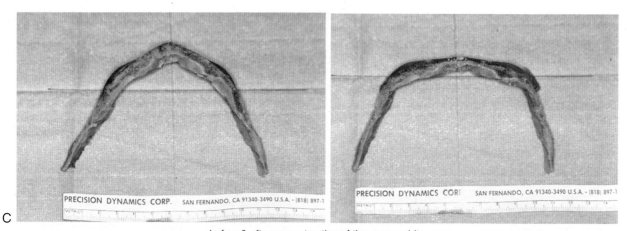

C   before & after reconstruction of the upper orbits

Figure 1.1, cont'd B, Illustrations of the craniofacial skeleton in a child with metopic synostosis resulting in trigonocephaly before and after anterior cranial vault and three-quarter orbital osteotomies. C, Bird's-eye view of removed orbital osteotomy unit prior to and after reshaping.

Continued

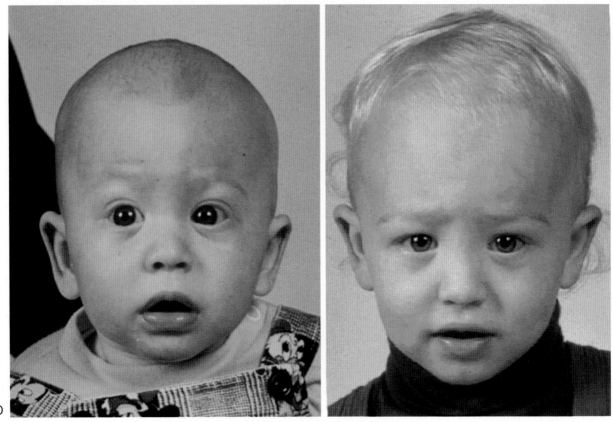

before & early after reconstruction

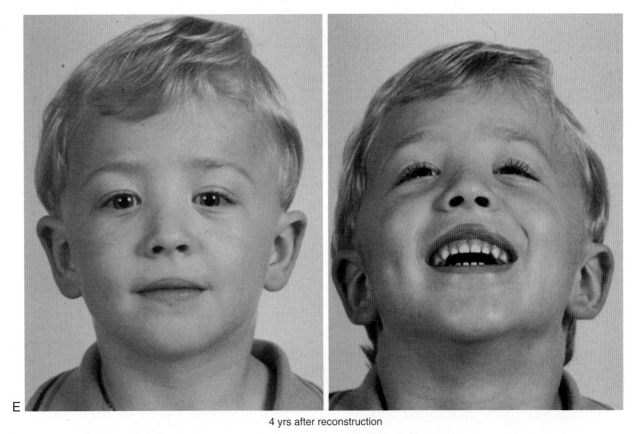

4 yrs after reconstruction

Figure 1.1, cont'd D, Frontal views before and 1 year after reconstruction. **E**, Facial views at 5 years of age.

Continued

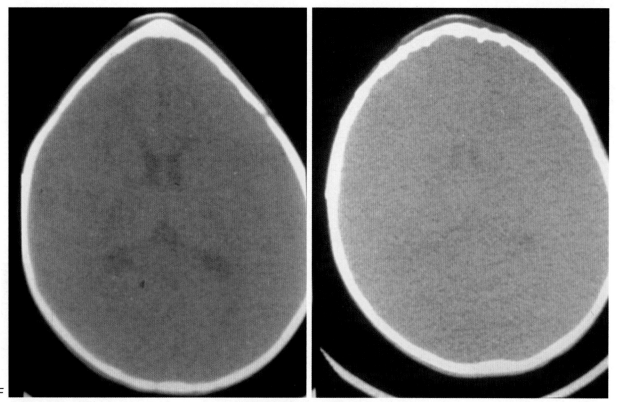

before & after reconstruction of the cranial vault and upper orbits

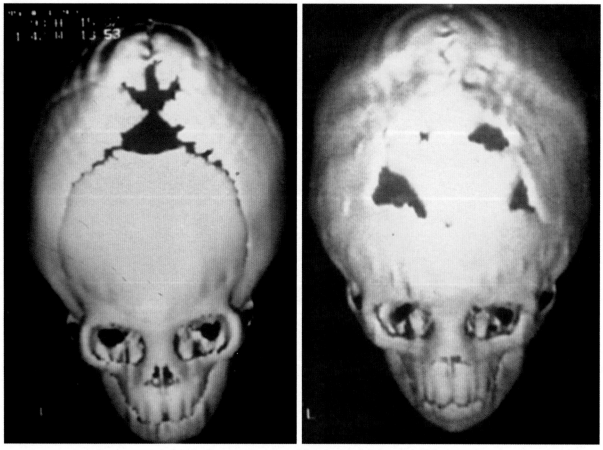

before & after reconstruction of the cranial vault & upper orbits

Figure 1.1, cont'd F and G, CT scan views before and after reconstruction. (A–G) From Posnick JC. Hereditary, developmental and environmental influences in the formation of dentofacial deformities. *Orthognathic Surgery: Principles and Practice,* 2nd ed. (JC Posnick, ed., B Kinard, assoc. ed.). St. Louis: Elsevier. Ch. 4, Fig. 4.20, pp. 112–13; 2022.

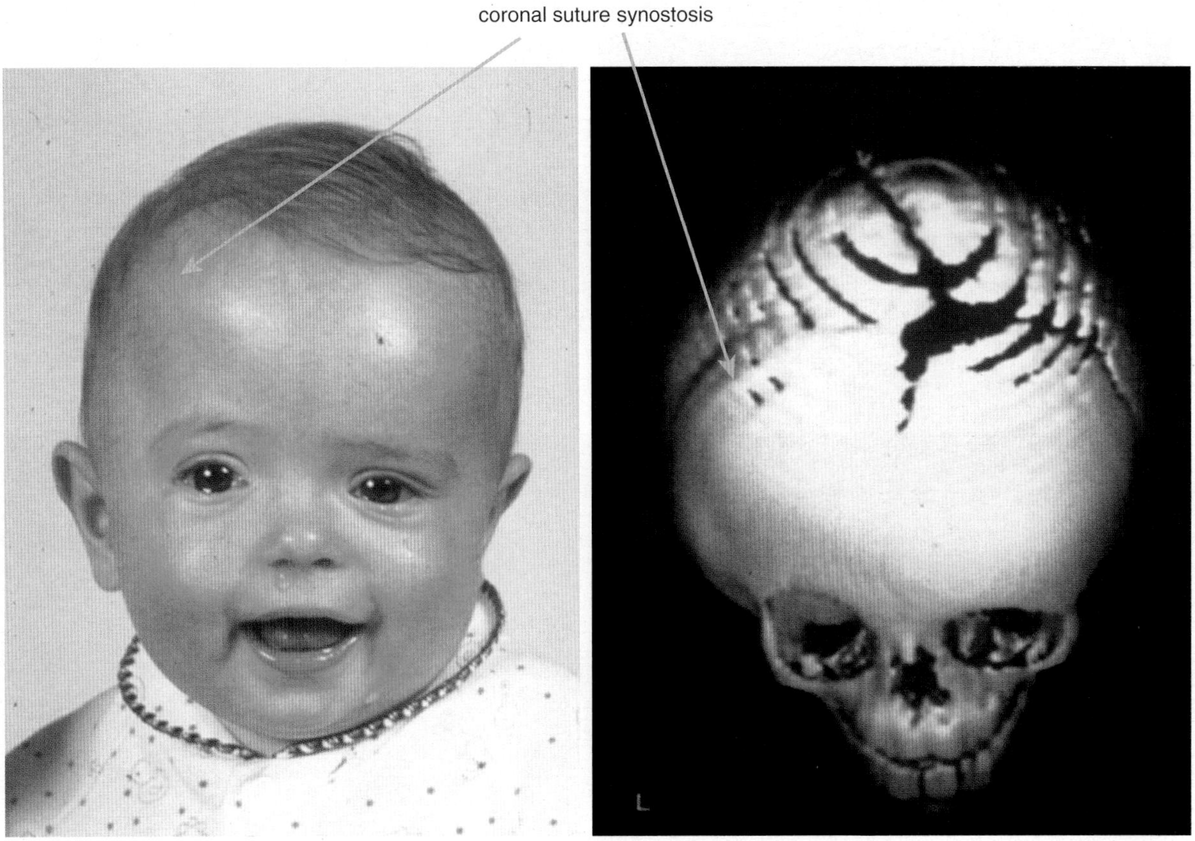

coronal suture synostosis

anterior plagiocephaly: caused by unilateral coronal suture synostosis

• **Figure 1.2** A child born with right unilateral coronal synostosis resulting in anterior plagiocephaly. He underwent anterior cranial vault and three-quarter orbital osteotomies with reshaping at 9 months of age. **A,** Facial and CT scan views prior to reconstruction.

Continued

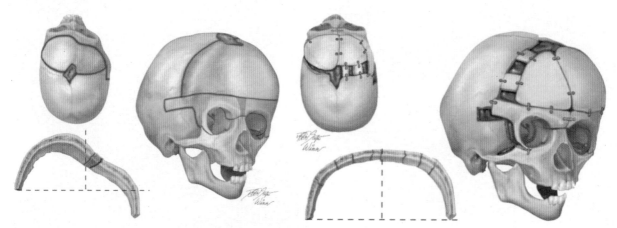

illustrations before & after reconstruction of the cranial vault & upper orbits

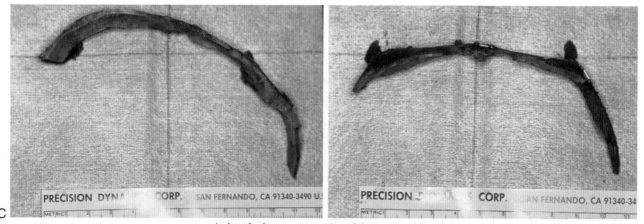

before & after reconstruction of the upper orbits

Figure 1.2, cont'd B, Illustrations of the craniofacial skeleton in a child with unilateral coronal synostosis resulting in anterior plagiocephaly before and after anterior cranial vault and three-quarter orbital osteotomies. **C,** Bird's-eye view of removed orbital osteotomy units prior to and after reshaping.

Continued

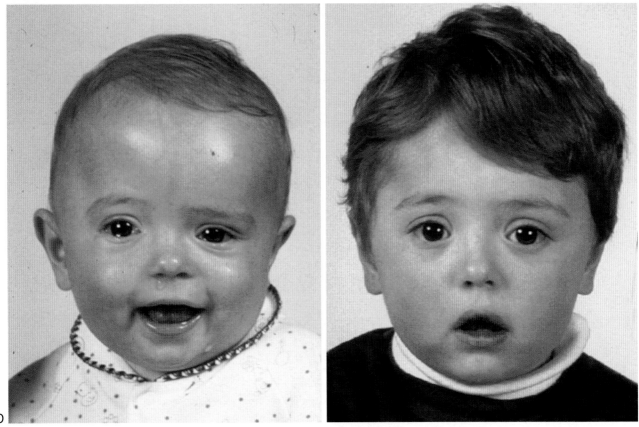

before & 4 yrs after reconstruction

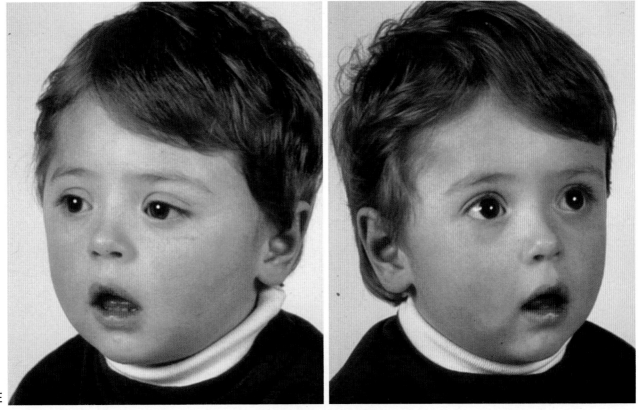

4 yrs after reconstruction

Figure 1.2, cont'd D, Frontal views before and 5 years after reconstruction. **E**, Oblique views 5 years after reconstruction.

Continued

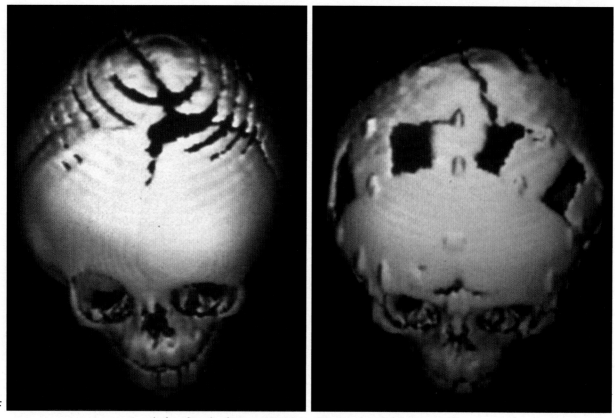

before & early after reconstruction of the cranial vault & upper orbits

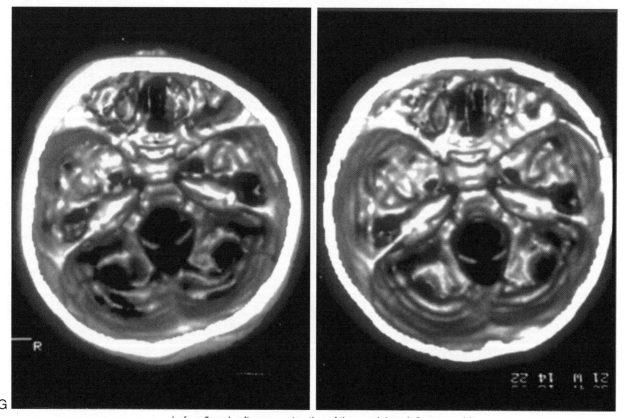

before & early after reconstruction of the cranial vault & upper orbits

Figure 1.2, cont'd F and G, CT scan views of cranial vault before and just after reconstruction. (A–G) From Posnick JC. Hereditary, developmental and environmental influences in the formation of dentofacial deformities. *Orthognathic Surgery: Principles and Practice*, 2nd ed. (JC Posnick, ed., B Kinard, assoc. ed.). St. Louis: Elsevier. Ch. 4, Fig. 4.21, pp. 114–16; 2022.

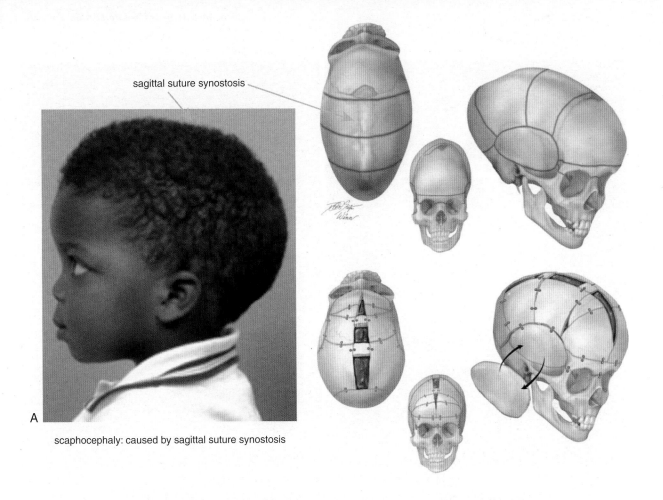

sagittal suture synostosis

A

scaphocephaly: caused by sagittal suture synostosis

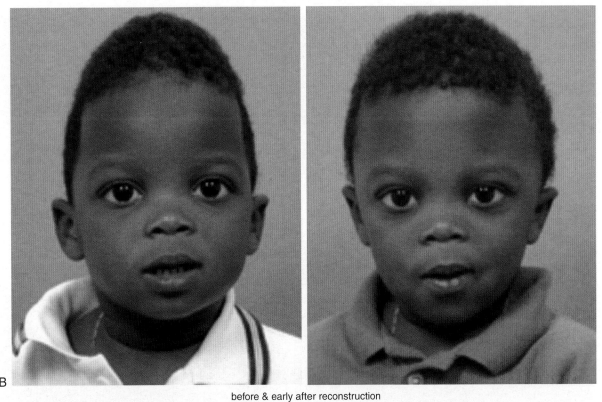

B

before & early after reconstruction

• **Figure 1.3** A child was born with sagittal synostosis resulting in a scaphocephalic shape to the cranial vault characterized by increased anterior–posterior length and decreased bi-temporal and bi-parietal width. It was not until 2 years of age that he was diagnosed with sagittal synostosis. After comprehensive evaluation, he underwent total cranial vault reshaping through a coronal (scalp) incision. He is shown before and after single-stage reconstruction. **A**, Profile facial view and illustrations of the craniofacial skeleton in a child with sagittal synostosis resulting in scaphocephaly, before and after total cranial vault and upper orbital osteotomies with reconstruction. **B**, Frontal facial views before and after reconstruction.

Continued

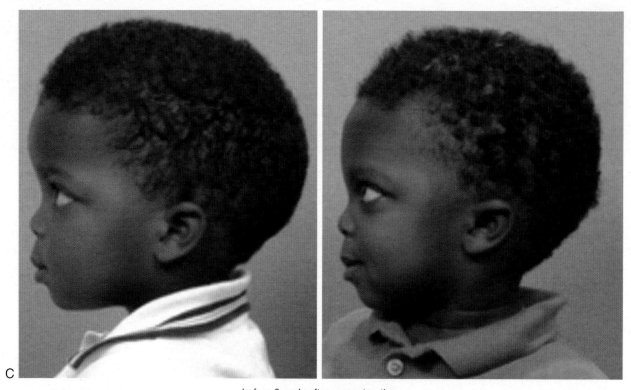

C

before & early after reconstruction

Figure 1.3, cont'd C, Profile facial views before and after reconstruction. (A–C) From Posnick JC. Hereditary, developmental and environmental influences in the formation of dentofacial deformities. *Orthognathic Surgery: Principles and Practice*, 2nd ed. (JC Posnick, ed., B Kinard, assoc. ed.). St. Louis: Elsevier. Ch. 4, Fig. 4.22, pp. 117–18; 2022.

References

1. Virchow R. Uber den Cretinismus, namentlich in Franken und uber pathologische Schadelformen. *Verh Phys Med GEs Wurzburg.* 1851;2:230.

2. Renier D, Sainte-Rose C, Marchac D, et al. Intracranial pressure in craniosynostosis. *J Neurosurg.* 1982;57:370.

3. Seruya M, Oh A, Boyajian M, Posnick JC, Keating R. Treatment for delayed presentation of sagittal synostosis: challenges pertaining to occult intracranial hypertension. *J Neurosurg-Pediatr.* 2011;8:40–48.

4. Tessier P, Guiot G, Rougerie J, et al. Osteotomies cranio-naso-orbito-faciales, hypertelorisme. *Chir Plast.* 1967;12:103.

5. Posnick JC, Lin KY, Chen P, Armstrong D. Sagittal synostosis: quantitative assessment of presenting deformity and surgical results based on CT scans. *Plast Reconstr Surg.* 1993;92(6):1015–1024.

6. Posnick JC, Lin KY, Chen P, Armstrong D. Metopic synostosis: quantitative assessment of presenting deformity and surgical results based on CT scans. *Plast Reconstr Surg.* 1994;93(1):16–24.

7. Utria A, Lopez J, Cho R, et al. Timing of cranial vault remodeling in non-syndromic craniosynostosis: a single institution's thirty-year experience. *J Neurosurg-Pediatr.* 2016;18:629–634.

8. Morrow BT, Ditthakasem K, Herbert M, Fearon JA. Perioperative outcomes following pediatric cranial vault remodeling: are improvements possible? *J Craniofac Surg.* 2019;30(7):2018–2022.

2

Reconstruction of Craniosynostosis Syndromes

JEFFREY C. POSNICK, DMD, MD

At birth, the skull, which is composed of multiple bones loosely connected by sutures, will have an expected "normal" shape and capacity for the underlying brain. "Open" sutures serve as growth centers for the cranial vault and actively stretch as the normal brain rapidly expands during infancy.[1] In embryologic life, if the bones of the skull directly connect without these expansile sutures (i.e., premature suture fusion) then growth of the cranial vault is inhibited (i.e., this is called craniosynostosis) (see Chapter 1). Craniosynostosis that also causes fusion of the skull base sutures will result in not just a compressed brain, but also in shallow orbits with bulging eyes, and a hypoplastic abnormal mid-facial appearance.[1] This is seen in syndromal forms of craniosynostosis.

The child's facial appearance, potential for brain and vision dysfunction, airway complications and chewing difficulties will be dependent on the particular combination of cranial vault and skull base premature suture line closures. Each common pattern of craniosynostosis that also affects the skull base sutures is considered a unique syndrome (i.e., craniosynostosis syndrome) and is often named after the doctor who first reported it to the literature, for example, Apert syndrome (see Fig. 2.1), named after Dr. Eugène Apert,[2] and Crouzon syndrome (see Fig. 2.2), named after Dr. Octave Crouzon.[3] Crouzon was the first to recognize a hereditary pattern for the observed set of malformations in a family with craniosynostosis. Based on the history of a family in Dorset, UK, Crouzon submitted a report to the medical literature in 1915. In Crouzon's report, the family members stated that "the deformities were present at birth and then accelerated during childhood". The deformities included: "a distinct hard ridge of the lower forehead"; "bulging eyes with impaired vision [e.g., strabismus and papilledema]"; "a prominent appearing lower jaw

with setback upper teeth [malocclusion] and a lower lip that protrudes" (see Fig. 2.2). Overall, the face [profile] was said to "resemble the appearance of the beak of a parrot [large appearing nose with setback jaw]". Unfortunately, other than documenting the findings, there was little that Crouzon could do to help alleviate the condition. The Dorset family was destined to a life of isolation, cognitive delay, seizures, loss of vision, and breathing difficulties.[3]

To limit brain compression, surgically releasing the fused skull sutures and expansion of the cranial vault can now be carried out during infancy (see Chapter 1). The surgery is to provide needed intracranial space (volume) to avoid damage to the infant's expanding brain.[1] Later in childhood, the residual cranial vault (skull) deformities, deficient orbits (i.e., the bones that surround the eyes), and midface hypoplasia (dished-in appearance of the upper jaw) should undergo definitive reconstruction through meticulously planned osteotomies and grafting procedures (i.e., frontofacial advancement) (see Figs. 2.1 and 2.2). The frontofacial advancement procedure performed later in childhood requires a transcranial approach, as innovated and pioneered by Dr. Paul Tessier over half a century ago.[4-6] During the teenage years, definitive jaw surgery coordinated with orthodontic treatment is required to complete the facial reconstruction (see Fig. 2.3).

The optimal surgery for a child born with a craniosynostosis syndrome continues to be discussed and undergo refinement, but the fundamental transcranial approach initially described by Tessier makes the reconstruction possible.[7-9] Unfortunately, even today most parents and caretakers of children born with a craniosynostosis syndrome still struggle to find a properly trained surgeon to bring about a successful facial reconstruction.

Letters from Past Patients

Dear Dr. Posnick,

I'm writing to thank you for all you have done for our daughter who was born with Crouzon syndrome. As you know, she went through a lot emotionally as a child with people staring at her. We as parents had a lot to learn as well when Sam was a baby and people would stare at us. You helped us get through an emotionally trying time in our life. It was unclear at the time if she would have brain damage and be developmentally delayed. As a result of the surgery this did not happen. Now in high school Sam is a straight-A student and has high goals for herself. Since the age of 6, she has set her lifetime ambition to be involved in the medical field. She hopes to be a craniofacial reconstructive surgeon one day.

Gratefully yours,
Gretchen and Stuart Porter

Dear Dr. Posnick,

This is a quick note to say hello. Just in case you don't remember us we have enclosed a few photographs of our daughter. We certainly remember you. Debbie is now in grade 10. She was born with Apert syndrome and the two facial surgeries that you performed changed our daughter's life. She is now doing well in school with good grades and is no longer being stared at. We are forever grateful.

Best wishes to you and your family,
Maryanne Wilson

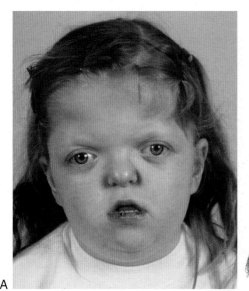

A

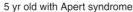

5 yr old with Apert syndrome

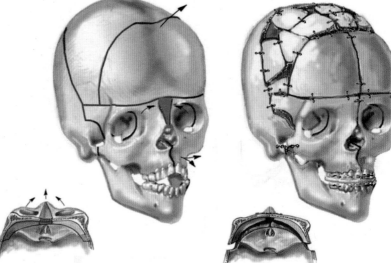

illustrations of cranial vault & facial bipartition reconstruction

• **Figure 2.1** A 5-year-old girl with Apert syndrome underwent initial cranial vault surgery when she was 6 months old and in the care of a neurosurgeon. She then presented to this surgeon with residual craniofacial deformities that required anterior cranial vault and facial bipartition (FB) osteotomies with reshaping and advancement (i.e., a type of frontofacial advancement). **A,** Facial view at 5 years of age and illustrations of preoperative craniofacial morphology and the planned cranial vault and FB reconstruction.

Continued

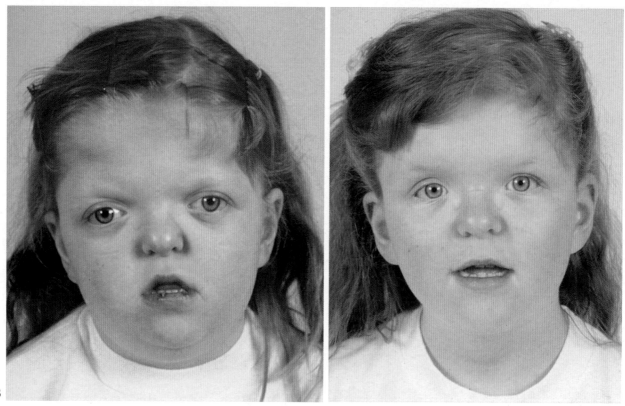

before & after cranial vault & facial bipartition reconstruction

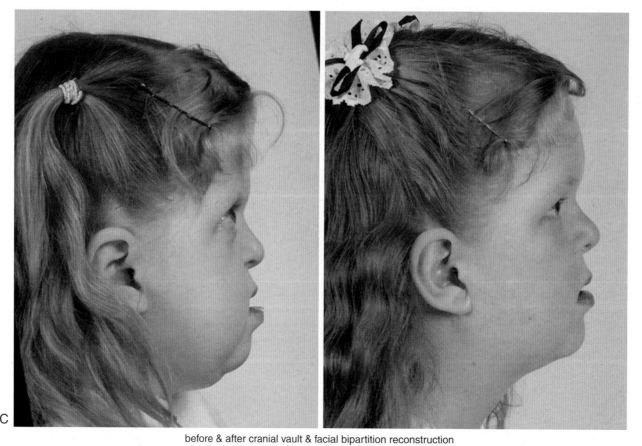

before & after cranial vault & facial bipartition reconstruction

Figure 2.1, cont'd **B,** Frontal facial views before and after FB reconstruction. **C,** Profile views before and after FB reconstruction.

Continued

bulging
eyes

normal
positioned
eyes

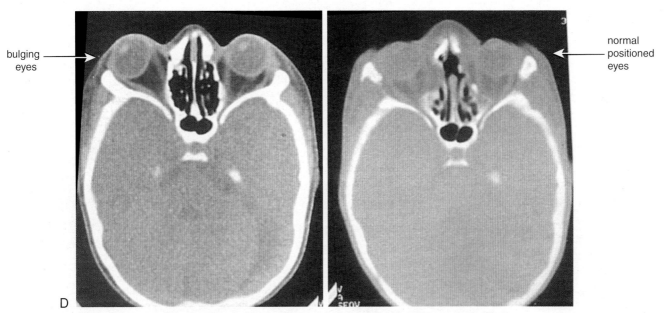

D

CT scan views before & after cranial vault & facial bipartition reconstruction

Figure 2.1, cont'd D, Computed tomography (CT) scan views through the midorbits before and after FB reconstruction that demonstrate improvement in orbital hypertelorism and orbital depth with diminished eye proptosis. (A–D) From Posnick JC. Crouzon syndrome: Evaluation and staging of reconstruction. *Craniofacial and Maxillofacial Surgery in Children and Young Adults* (JC Posnick, ed.). Philadelphia: W.B. Saunders Co. Ch. 14, pp. 271–307; 2000.

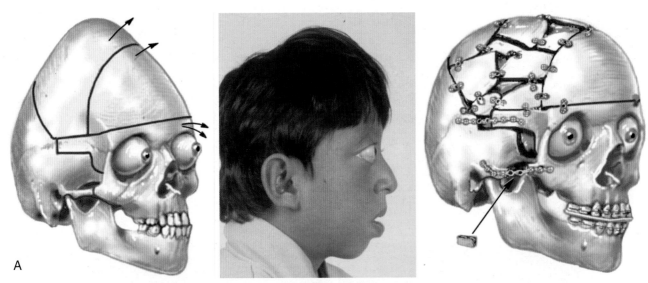

A

12 yr old with Crouzon syndrome illustrations before & after fronto-facial reconstruction

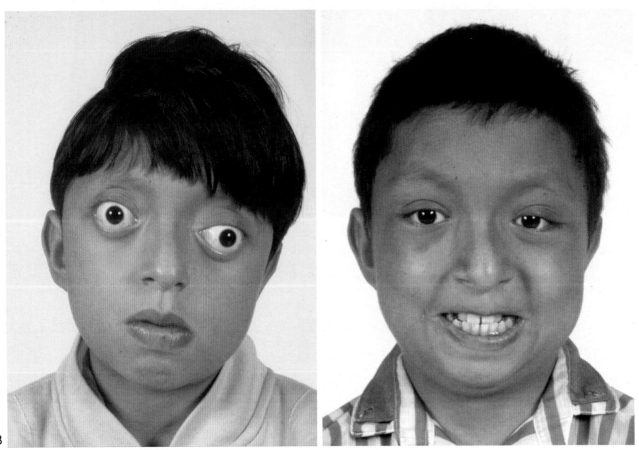

B

before & after fronto-facial advancement reconstruction

• **Figure 2.2** A 12-year-old boy with unrepaired Crouzon syndrome was referred to this surgeon for evaluation. He had not undergone any previous interventions. He underwent total cranial vault and monobloc (MB) osteotomies with advancement (i.e., a type of frontofacial advancement). **A,** Profile facial view before surgery. Illustrations of the patient's craniofacial morphology with planned cranial vault and MB osteotomy locations and then after completion. **B,** Facial views before and after MB reconstruction.

Continued

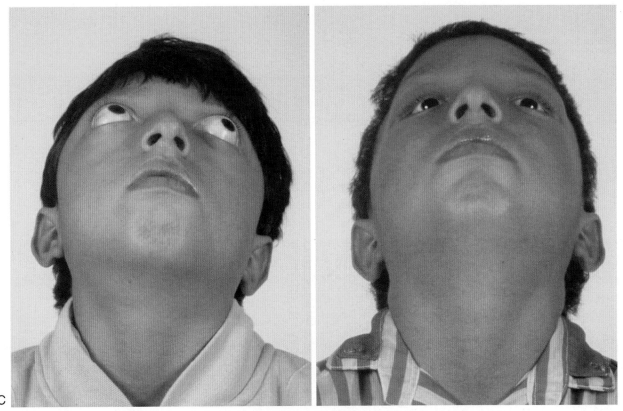

before & after fronto-facial advancement reconstruction

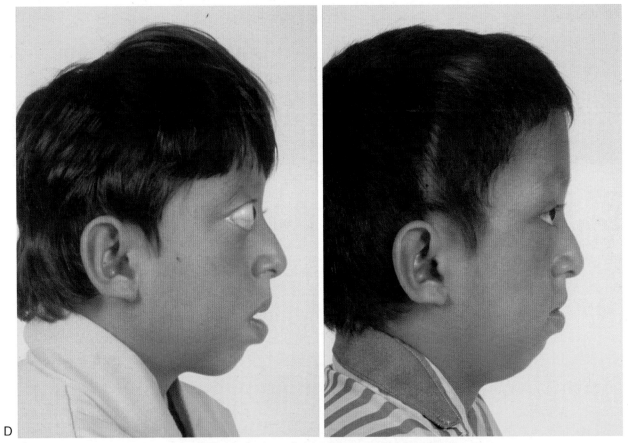

before & after fronto-facial advancement reconstruction

Figure 2.2, cont'd **C,** Worm's-eye views before and after MB reconstruction. **D,** Profile views before and after MB reconstruction.

Continued

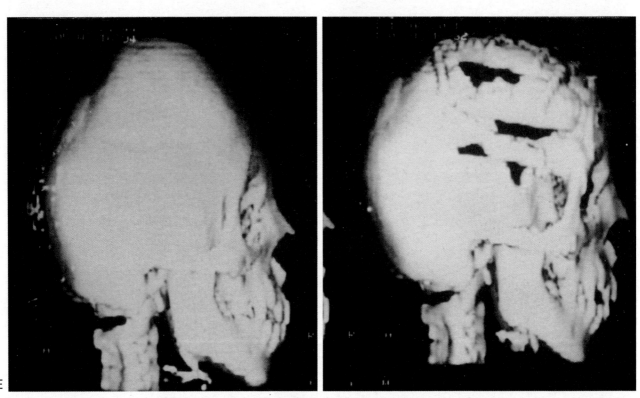

CT scan views before & after fronto-facial advancement reconstruction

Figure 2.2, cont'd **E,** CT scan views before and immediately after reconstruction. (A–E) From Posnick JC. Crouzon syndrome: Evaluation and staging of reconstruction. *Craniofacial and Maxillofacial Surgery in Children and Young Adults* (JC Posnick, ed.). Philadelphia: W.B. Saunders Co. Ch. 14, pp. 271–307; 2000.

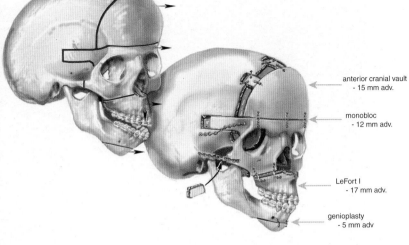

14 yrs of age with Crouzon syndrome   illustrations of cranial vault, fronto-facial advancement & jaw reconstruction

anterior cranial vault
- 15 mm adv.

monobloc
- 12 mm adv.

LeFort I
- 17 mm adv.

genioplasty
- 5 mm adv

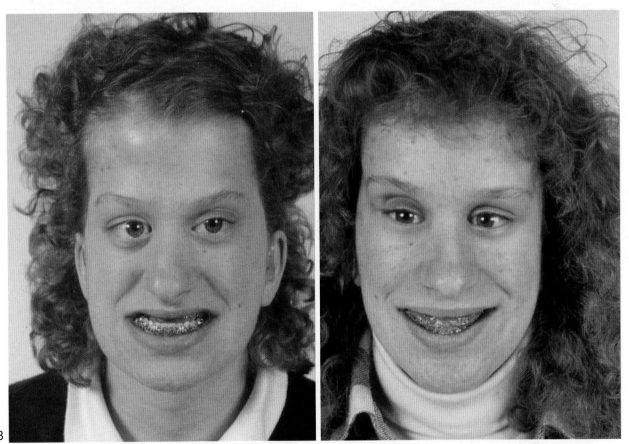

before & after fronto-facial & jaw reconstruction

• **Figure 2.3** A child who was born with Crouzon syndrome underwent bilateral coronal suture release when she was 3 months old. This was followed by additional cranial vault reshaping when she was 9 months old. At 2 years of age she underwent a transcranial Le Fort III midface osteotomy and additional forehead advancement. She presented to this surgeon when she was 14 years of age with residual deformity for which she underwent simultaneous single-stage anterior cranial vault, frontofacial (MB), Le Fort I, and chin osteotomies. **A,** Profile facial view at 14 years of age and illustrations of planned and completed anterior cranial vault, frontofacial (MB), Le Fort I, and chin osteotomies. **B,** Frontal facial views before and after definitive reconstruction.

Continued

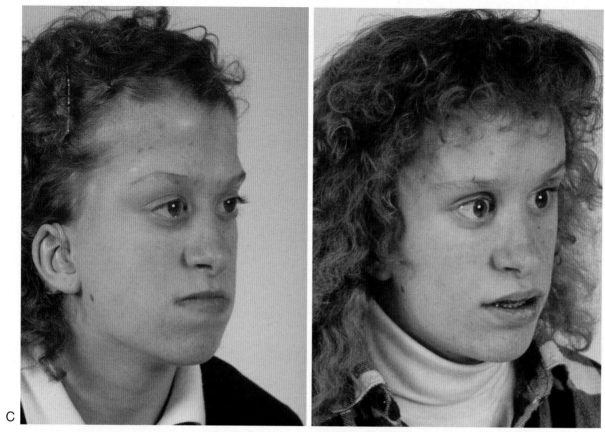

before & after fronto-facial & jaw reconstruction

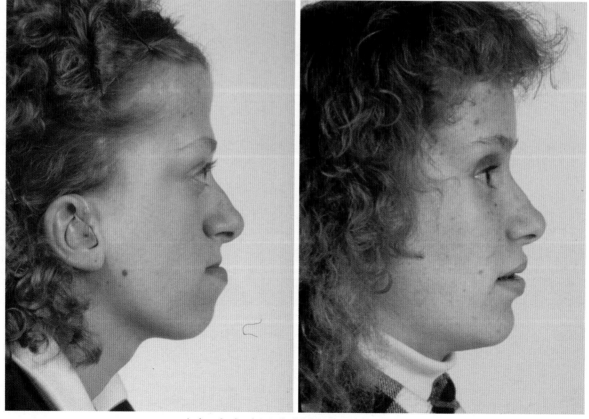

before & after fronto-facial & jaw reconstruction

Figure 2.3, cont'd **C,** Oblique facial views before and after definitive reconstruction. **D,** Profile views before and after definitive reconstruction.

Continued

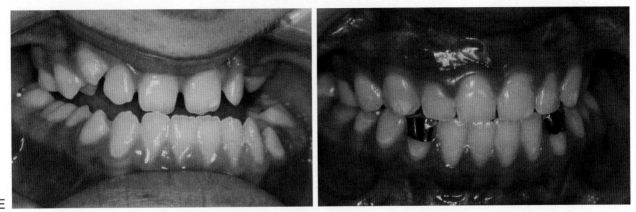

E

occlusal views before & after fronto-facial & jaw reconstruction

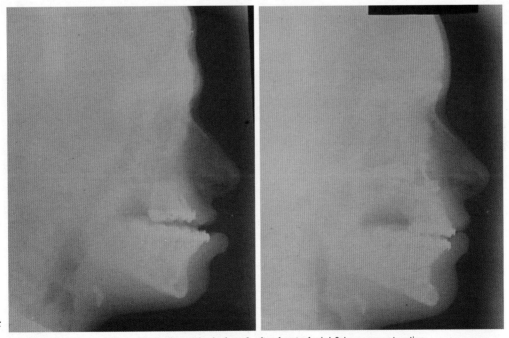

F

cephalometric radiographs before & after fronto-facial & jaw reconstruction

Figure 2.3, cont'd E, Occlusal views before and after reconstruction and orthodontic treatment. F, Lateral cephalometric radiographs before and after reconstruction.

Continued

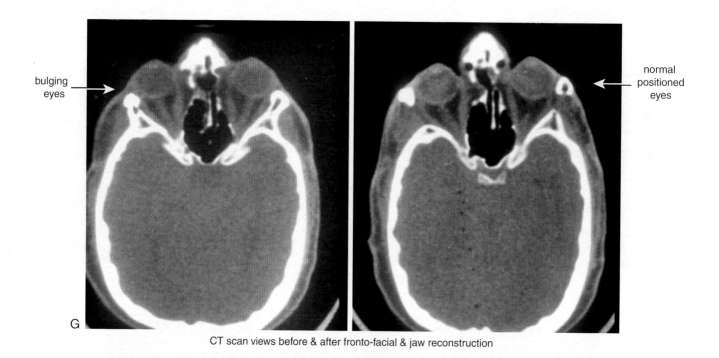

bulging
eyes

normal
positioned
eyes

CT scan views before & after fronto-facial & jaw reconstruction

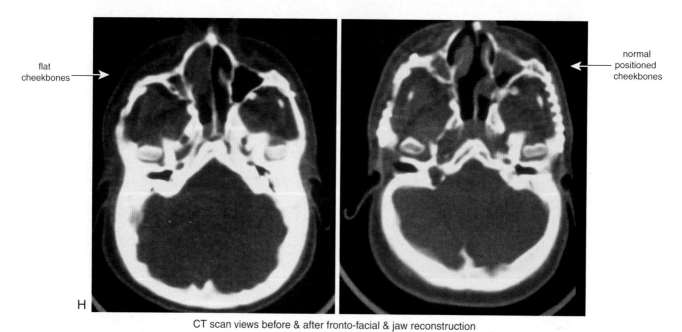

flat
cheekbones

normal
positioned
cheekbones

CT scan views before & after fronto-facial & jaw reconstruction

Figure 2.3, cont'd **G,** Axial CT scan views through the midorbits before and after reconstruction confirms relief of proptosis. **H,** Axial CT scan views through the zygomatic arches before and after reconstruction confirms improved cheekbone projection. (A–H) From Posnick JC. Crouzon syndrome: Evaluation and staging of reconstruction. *Craniofacial and Maxillofacial Surgery in Children and Young Adults* (JC Posnick, ed.). Philadelphia: W.B. Saunders Co. Ch. 14, pp. 288–291; 2000.

References

1. Cohen Jr MM. Apert, Crouzon, and Pfeiffer syndromes. In: Muenke M, Kress W, Collmann H, Solomon BD, eds. *Craniosynostoses: Molecular Genetics, Diagnosis, and Treatment.* Vol. 19. Basle: Karger; 2011:67–88. Monographs in Human Genetics.

2. Apert E. De l'acrocephalosyndactlie. *Bull Mem Soc Med Hop Paris.* 1906;23:1310.

3. Crouzon O. Une nouvelle famille atteinte de dysostose craniofaciale hereditaire. *Arch Med Enfants.* 1915;18:540.

4. Tessier P. Total facial osteotomy. Crouzon syndrome, Apert syndrome: oxycephaly, scaphocephaly, turricephaly. [French] *Ann Chir Plast.* 1967;12:273–286.

5. Tessier P. The definitive plastic surgical treatment of the severe facial deformities of craniofacial synostosis: Crouzon and Apert diseases. *Plast Reconstr Surg.* 1971;48:419.

6. Tessier P. The monobloc and frontofacial advancement: do the pluses outweigh the minuses? [discussion]. *Plast Reconstr Surg.* 1993;91:988.

7. Posnick JC, Al-Qattan MM, Armstrong D. Monobloc and facial bipartition osteotomies: quantitative assessment of presenting deformity and surgical results based on computed tomography scans. *J Oral Maxillofac Surg.* 1995;53:358–367.

8. Posnick JC. Monobloc and facial bipartition osteotomies: a step-by-step description of the surgical technique. *J Craniofac Surg.* 1996;7(3):229–250.

9. Posnick JC. Syndromes with craniosynostosis: evaluation and treatment. In: Posnick JC, ed., Kinard B, assoc. ed. *Orthognathic Surgery: Principles and Practice.* 2nd ed. St. Louis: Elsevier; 2022. ch. 30.

3

Reconstruction of Complex Facial Clefts

JEFFREY C. POSNICK, DMD, MD

During embryological development the two halves of the face start out separated from each other at the midline. By 5–8 weeks of embryologic life, in almost all fetuses, the facial halves meet and join together perfectly. On occasion, the facial halves remain partially (i.e., limited midline nasal clefting) or completely (i.e., complete midline facial clefting) separated at birth. When complete midline facial clefting occurs, negative effects on the child's vision, feeding ability, and speech are to be expected. The child's facial appearance will also be strikingly abnormal and will warrant attention as soon as feasible.

In the late 1960s, Dr. Paul Tessier demonstrated how the forehead and midfacial skeleton, in a child with congenital deformity, could be surgically disassembled and then reconstructed while working through a transcranial approach.[1] It was only after years of work perfecting the technique of intracranial reconstruction that Tessier presented his novel approach to manage complex facial deformities and skull base tumors. His initial presentation was at an international medical meeting in Rome in 1966.[2] The surgeons in attendance were in disbelief and there was an uproar that the techniques were unproven and much too dangerous. Tessier offered to perform live surgery at the Hôpital Foch in Paris under the observation of a panel of experts to let them judge. After attending the procedures, the panelists were asked to either vote in favor of his continued work or denial, in which case he would agree to immediately stop. After a resounding vote of confidence by an astonished group of surgeons, patients around the world were given hope for the removal of previously incurable tumors, for the management of complex facial fractures, and for relief from disabling congenital malformations.[3] Tessier's innovations continue to allow surgeons cranial base access for the removal of tumors and to safely reconstruct all the facial bones.

In 1979, Dr. Jacques Van der Meulen, of Rotterdam, further innovated on Tessier's transcranial approach by suggesting that after surgically separating the facial bones from the skull base, the freed-up skeleton could be split down the midline and then positioned closer together for reconstruction.[4] After additional technical refinements were introduced, remarkable reconstructions for children with midline facial clefting became possible (see Figs. 3.1 and 3.2).[6,7]

As midline facial clefting is rare, few surgeons develop the expertise to safely correct the affected child's functional needs (i.e., vision, speech, chewing) and to achieve an optimal facial appearance that is then maintained into adulthood.[5–7] In the future, it is hoped that molecular geneticists will be able to predict and alter these anomalies in utero. If not, when these malformations do occur, advanced technology will improve the precision of reconstruction without as much reliance on the individual surgeon's personal skill set.

Letter from a Past Patient (see Fig. 3.2)

Dear Dr. Posnick,

I don't know if you remember me, but I was a patient of yours when I was a child. I was born with my face split down the middle and you completed my facial reconstructive surgery. I've been wanting to write to you for a long time now and say thank you! You changed my life immensely. I now have a five-year-old son. I have included a photograph of us and as you can see, he is without the same problem. You will always be part of our life.

Yours truly,
Courtney Livingston

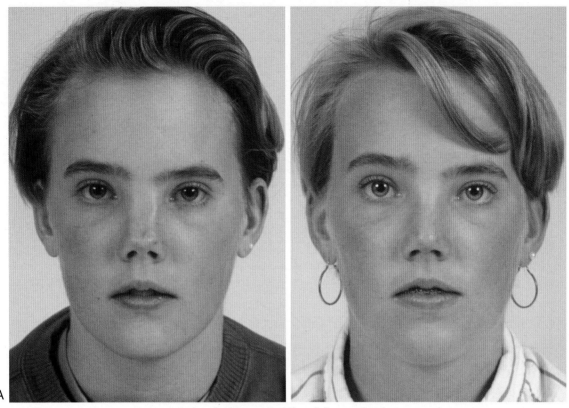

before & after nasal midline cleft reconstruction

A

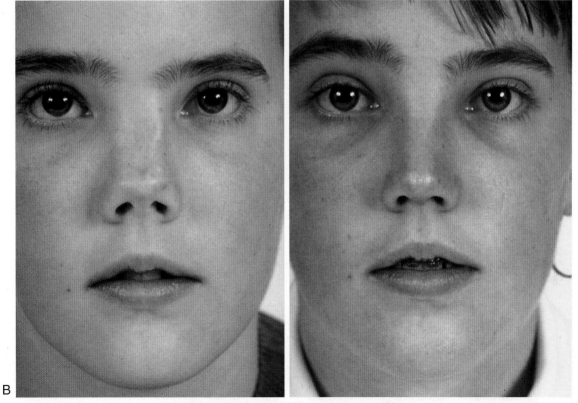

before & after nasal midline cleft reconstruction

B

• **Figure 3.1** A 15-year-old girl born with a mild Tessier 0 and 14 craniofacial cleft. There is congenital separation of the nasal bones and the septum. The degree of orbital hypertelorism (i.e., separation of the eyes) is minimal. She underwent reconstruction that included nasal osteotomies and augmentation of the dorsum of the nose (from the radix to the tip) with a crafted and rigidly fixated full-thickness cranial bone graft. The lower lateral cartilages were sutured over the top of the cranial graft to create the new nasal tip. Access was gained through coronal scalp and open rhinoplasty (columella splitting) incisions. **A,** Frontal views before and after reconstruction. **B,** Close-up frontal view of the nose before and after reconstruction.

Continued

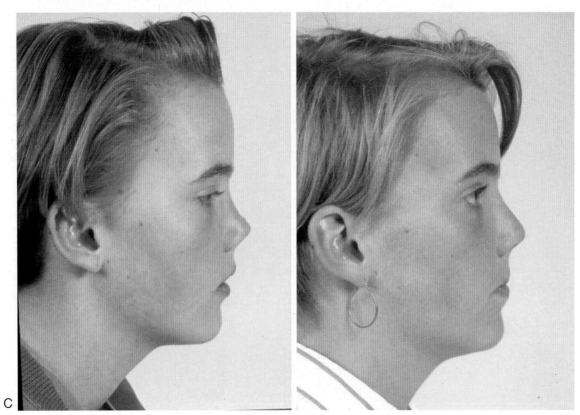

before & after nasal midline cleft reconstruction

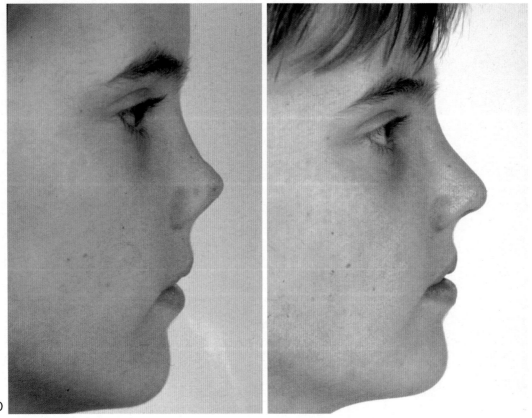

before & after midline nasal cleft reconstruction

Figure 3.1, cont'd C, Profile views of nose before and after reconstruction. **D,** Close-up profile view of nose before and after reconstruction.
Continued

bone graft in place at junction of nose & forehead

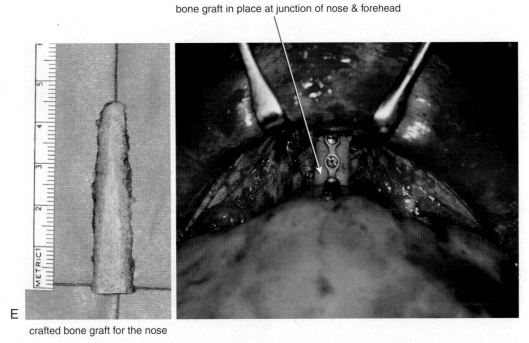

E

crafted bone graft for the nose

Figure 3.1, cont'd E, Intraoperative view of crafted full-thickness cranial graft (45 mm in length). View of the frontonasal region with a rigidly fixated graft to create the correct nasofrontal angle. (A–E) From Posnick JC. Rare facial clefts: Evaluation and treatment. *Craniofacial and Maxillofacial Surgery in Children and Young Adults* (JC Posnick, ed.). Philadelphia: W.B. Saunders Co. Ch. 23, pp. 487–502; 2000.

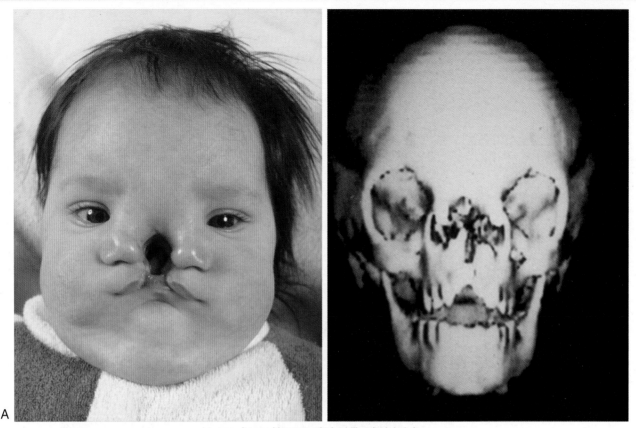

newborn with congenital midline facial cleft

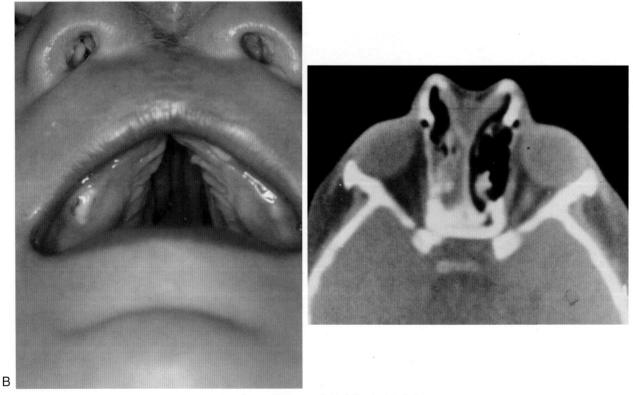

newborn with congenital midline facial cleft

• **Figure 3.2** A child born with a complex midline facial cleft. She underwent repair of the cleft lip when she was 1 year old; this was followed by cleft palate closure when she was 18 months old at another institution. She was referred to this surgeon at 4 years of age for craniofacial reconstruction. She underwent a bifrontal craniotomy and facial bipartition (FB) osteotomies. The two halves of the face were then three-dimensionally repositioned for the correction of upper-face hypertelorism and to close the cleft of the nose and the upper jaw. **A,** Facial and computed tomography (CT) scan views early after birth. **B,** Facial and CT scan views after lip repair but before palate closure.

Continued

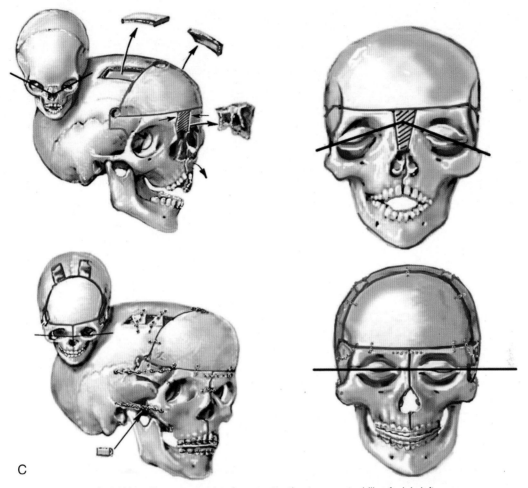

C

facial bipartition osteotomies & reconstruction to correct midline facial cleft

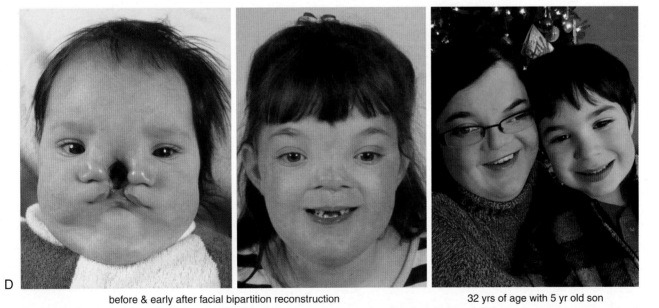

D

before & early after facial bipartition reconstruction   32 yrs of age with 5 yr old son

Figure 3.2, cont'd C, Illustrations of the craniofacial skeleton with proposed and completed anterior cranial vault and FB osteotomies and reconstruction. **D,** Facial views before and after reconstruction. She is also shown at 32 years of age (28 years after reconstruction) with her 5-year-old son. (A–D) From Posnick JC. Rare facial clefts: evaluation and treatment. *Craniofacial and Maxillofacial Surgery in Children and Young Adults* (JC Posnick, ed.). Philadelphia: W.B. Saunders Co. Ch. 23, pp. 487–502; 2000.

References

1. Tessier P. The definitive plastic surgical treatment of the severe facial deformities of craniofacial synostosis: crouzon and Apert diseases. *Plast Reconstr Surg*. 1971;48:419.

2. Tessier P. Dysostosis cranio-faciales (syndromes de Crouzon et d'Apert) osteotomies totales de la face. *Transactions of the Fourth International Congress of Plastic and Reconstructive Surgery, Rome, 1967*. Amsterdam: Excerpta Medica Foundation; 1969:774–783.

3. Tessier P. *Demonstration Operations at Hôpital Foch*. Paris: Suresnes; 1967.

4. Van der Meulen JC. Medial fasciotomy. *Br J Plast Surg*. 1979;32:339–342.

5. Tessier P. The monobloc and frontofacial advancement: do the pluses outweigh the minuses? [discussion]. *Plast Reconstr Surg*. 1993;91:988.

6. Posnick JC, Al-Qattan MM, Armstrong D. Monobloc and facial bipartition osteotomies: quantitative assessment of presenting deformity and surgical results based on computed tomography scans. *J Oral Maxillofac Surg*. 1995;53:358–367.

7. Posnick JC. Syndromes with craniosynostosis: evaluation and treatment. In: Posnick JC, ed., Kinard B, assoc. ed. *Orthognathic Surgery: Principles and Practice*. 2nd ed. St. Louis: Elsevier; 2022. ch. 30.

4
Reconstruction of Skull Defects

JEFFREY C. POSNICK, DMD, MD

The reconstruction of skull defects in children is warranted to protect the brain as well as for morphologic and body image concerns. Skull defects may occur as part of a larger malformation present since birth but are more commonly seen as a result of trauma to the cranial vault with loss of structure or as a consequence of tumor removal.

A skull defect reconstruction should provide functional protection to the brain and a normal cranial vault contour with minimal procedural risks. Over the past decades, numerous techniques, using a variety of materials to repair skull defects, have been described in the medical literature. For now, the use of the child's own adjacent uninjured skull bone, which is then split into inner and outer layers, as initially described by Tessier in the 1970s, remains the preferred method of reconstruction, when feasible.[1] The surgery requires intracranial access with the assistance of a neurosurgeon. For reconstruction of a skull defect, the surgically removed segment of intact (normal) cranial vault is then split into inner and outer layers, effectively doubling the surface area of bone with which to work.[2] The monocortical (single layer) bone grafts are then contoured and rigidly fixated in their new locations with specially designed hardware to minimize healing difficulties. The "one layer" cranial vault reconstruction at both the donor and recipient sites, while not as strong as nature had given, provides safe enough protection to the brain and restores normal morphology and shape to the head (see Figs. 4.1 and 4.2).[3]

After successful initial cranial vault healing, the return to most sports activities with a requirement for just the usual extent of head and face protection is typical. The cranial vault reconstruction should last a lifetime.[4] Unfortunately, the ideal artificial material for the definitive repair of skull defects in children and adults has yet to be developed.

The recent advent of computer-designed, patient-specific, three-dimensional implants will continue to revolutionize cranial defect reconstruction. Even in experienced hands, manual restoration of normal surface skull morphology is challenging. In the future, computer-aided design and computer-aided manufacturing technology will facilitate more accurate restoration of the missing skull components. This technology will become commonplace for use in both autogenous and alloplastic reconstruction worldwide.

Letter from a Past Patient

Hi Dr. Posnick,

Before we met you and Dr. Hendricks, we thought that our daughter would have to continue wearing a helmet for the rest of her life. The hole in her skull was so large you could feel the brain. We still marvel that because of the surgery that you did her head is now strong and she can play outside just like other children. We can't thank you enough.

God bless,
The Higgins family

infected methyl methacrylate cranioplasty

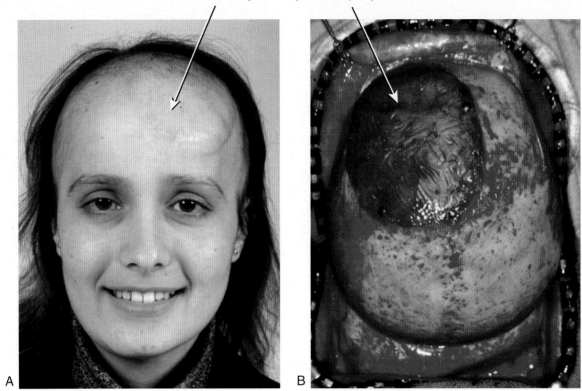

16 yr old with skull defect & radiation damaged scalp

infected methyl methacrylate removed

cranial graft cranioplasty

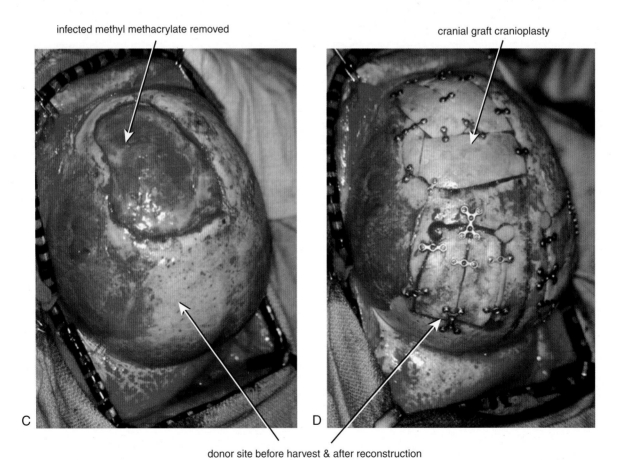

donor site before harvest & after reconstruction

• **Figure 4.1** A 16-year-old girl underwent intracranial resection of an astrocytoma located in the frontal lobe of the brain, followed by radiation therapy. Loss of the frontal bone flap followed by a methylmethacrylate (i.e., artificial material) cranioplasty resulted in recurrent cellulitis. She was then referred for evaluation. An autogenous cranial bone cranioplasty and soft tissue expansion (i.e., temporary placement of tissue expanders) of the posterior hair-bearing scalp was carried out, followed by resection of radiated forehead skin and posterior flap advancement of hair-bearing scalp to create a new anterior hairline. **A,** Facial view before removal of infected methylmethacrylate and before autogenous bone cranioplasty. **B,** Intraoperative view of cranial vault after elevation of coronal scalp flap. Note: methylmethacrylate cranioplasty not yet removed. **C,** View of cranial vault after removal of methylmethacrylate. **D,** Full-thickness cranial bone was harvested from the left and right occipital regions, split into inner and outer layers, and then used for reconstruction of donor and recipient sites.

Continued

tissue expander is under "expanded" scalp

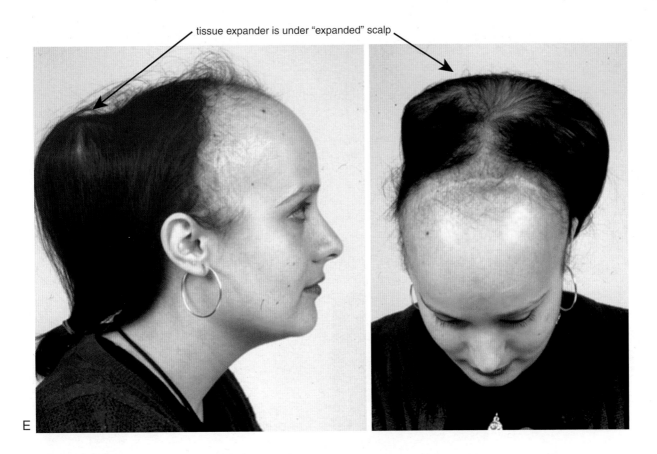

E

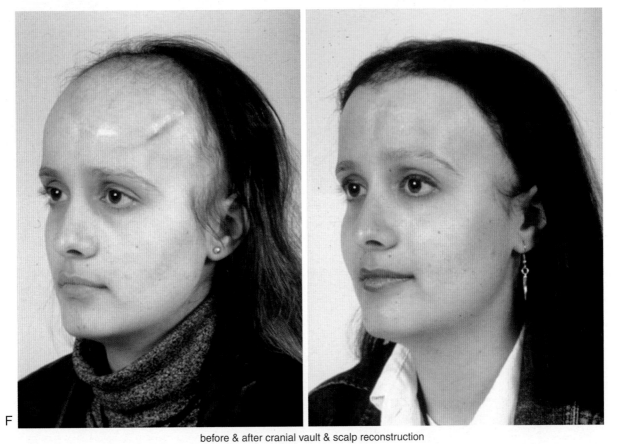

F

before & after cranial vault & scalp reconstruction

Figure 4.1, cont'd **E,** Views of "expanded" hair-bearing posterior scalp just prior to flap advancement reconstruction of a new anterior hairline.

Continued

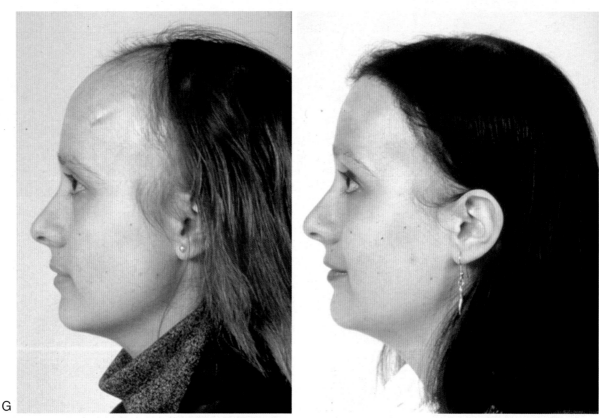

G

before & after cranial vault & scalp reconstruction

Figure 4.1, cont'd **F and G,** Oblique and profile facial views before and after reconstruction. (A–G) From Posnick JC. Sarcomas and other malignant head and neck tumors of childhood. *Craniofacial and Maxillofacial Surgery in Children and Young Adults* (JC Posnick, ed.). Philadelphia: W.B. Saunders Co. Ch. 28, pp. 620–654; 2000.

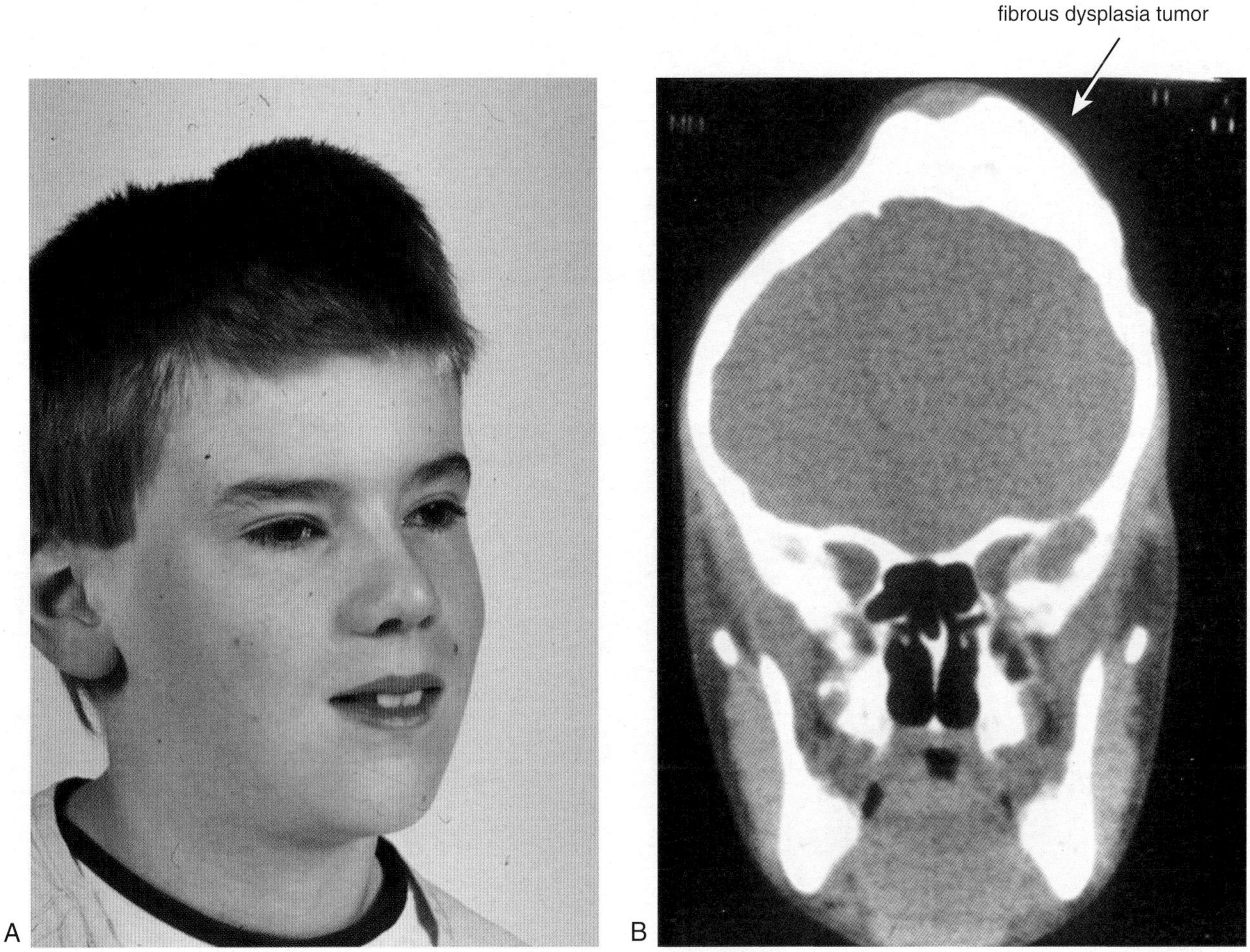

fibrous dysplasia tumor

A

B

10 yr old with tumor of the skull

• **Figure 4.2** A 10-year-old boy initially underwent incomplete excision of an expansive bone tumor (i.e., fibrous dysplasia) of the frontotemporal region at 2 years of age. The defect was initially reconstructed with rib grafts by another surgeon. The patient was referred to this surgeon for evaluation at 10 years of age with a large recurrent bony tumor. He underwent resection and immediate reconstruction with autogenous cranial bone grafts. **A,** Facial view at time of consultation. **B,** Computed tomography (CT) scan view through cranial vault demonstrating recurrent tumor.

Continued

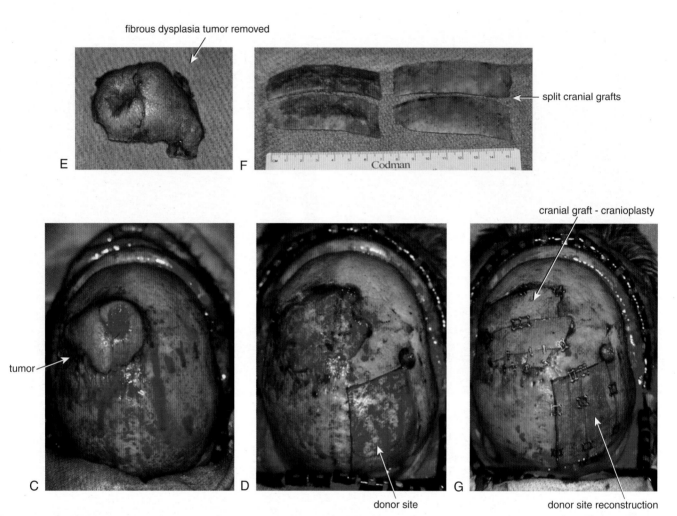

Figure 4.2, cont'd C, Intraoperative view of cranial vault before tumor resection. **D,** Intraoperative view after resection of tumor and harvesting of right parietal bone for reconstruction. **E,** Resected specimen is shown. **F,** Full-thickness cranial grafts have been split into inner and outer layers for reconstruction. **G,** View of reconstructed donor and recipient sites with fixated split cranial grafts.

Continued

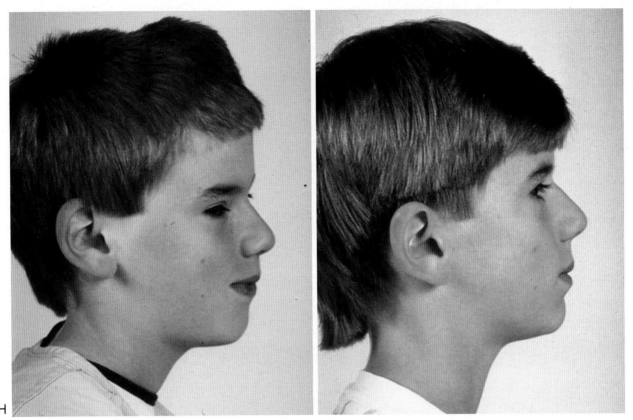

before & after tumor resection & reconstruction

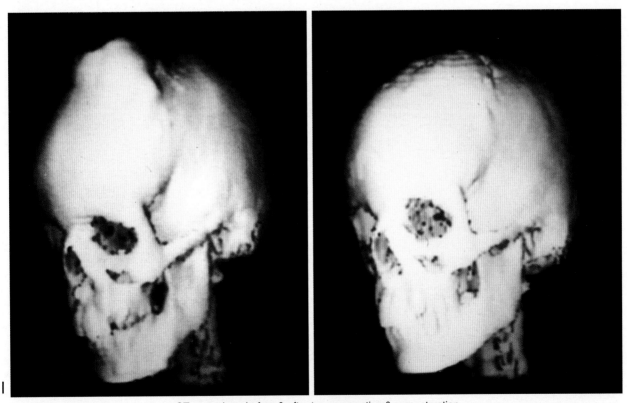

CT scan views before & after tumor resection & reconstruction

Figure 4.2, cont'd H, Profile views before and after resection and reconstruction. **I,** Comparison of 3-D CT scan views demonstrating bone tumor before and 1 year after resection/reconstruction. (A–I) From Posnick JC, Goldstein JA, Armstrong D, Rutka JT. Reconstruction of skull defects in children and adolescents by the use of fixed cranial bone grafts: Long-term results. *Neurosurgery*. 1993;32:785.

References

1. Tessier P. Autogenous bone grafts taken from the calvarium for facial and cranial applications. *Clin Plast Surg*. 1982;9:531.

2. Tessier P, Kawamoto H, Matthews D, et al. Taking calvarial grafts– tools and techniques: VI. The splitting of a parietal bone "flap". *Plast Reconstr Surg*. 2005;116(5):74S.

3. Posnick JC, Goldstein JA, Armstrong D, Rutka JT. Reconstruction of skull defects in children and adolescents by the use of fixed cranial bone grafts: long-term results. *J Neurosurg*. 1993;32(5):785–791.

4. Posnick JC. Management of secondary jaw deformities after maxillofacial trauma. In: Posnick JC, ed., Kinard B, assoc. ed. *Orthognathic Surgery: Principles and Practice*. 2nd ed. St. Louis: Elsevier; 2022. ch. 35.

5

Management of Congenital Tumors of the Face

JEFFREY C. POSNICK, DMD, MD

A non-malignant expansive tumor present at birth can distort normal embryologic growth and alter the morphology and function of the involved facial structures that are being compressed or expanded.[1] Frequent examples of congenital tumors that involve the face and cause significant deformities and malfunction include neurofibromatosis, vascular malformations, fibrous dysplasia, and congenital (neo-cellular) nevi.[2] The tumor mass may compress visceral structures (i.e. brain, eyes, ears) and cavities (i.e. throat, nose and sinus) thereby causing impairment of function. Depending on the tumor's location, volume, and velocity of growth, there may be alterations in the child's cognitive function, vision, speech, breathing, swallowing, chewing, lip control, hearing, neck, or mandibular range of motion.[3]

Decisions concerning the appropriate age for tumor removal in the child involve a delicate balance that takes into account: imminent functional needs (e.g., blindness, hearing deficit, massive bleeding, airway compromise); potential for malignant transformation; the safety of surgery at a young age; unique psychosocial concerns of the family; the residual facial growth requirements of the involved structures; and the secondary effects of early age surgery on facial development (see Figs. 5.1–5.6). With these unusual congenital tumors, each child's unique needs influence the surgeon's and family's decision concerning the age at which to operate and the extent of the procedure.[4] Decisions are often based on the surgeon's personal skills, experience, and comfort level with the procedures under consideration.[5] In the future, standardized protocols, based on the best scientific knowledge of the natural progression of these congenital growths, will direct treatment and improve outcomes.

Letters from Past Patients

Dear Dr. Posnick,

We have never met as we are the grandparents of Michael. When Michael was about 11 years old, he was watching a movie and he wanted me to sit with him and watch the whole film again. The name of the show was "The Elephant Man". At the end of the movie he said, "Mama this is me, this is how I feel." It's easy for you to understand this situation after you have taken care of so many children with similar problems but for me that day was so very sad. Now that you have helped Michael with his reconstructive surgery, this is no longer a problem for him.

Thank you so much.
Margaret and Ted Long

Dear Dr. Posnick,

I want to thank you for saving my son's life with your facial surgery for his tumor. Your expertise was much appreciated, and he is now doing very well.

Gratefully yours, blessings and peace,
Norah Miller

Hi Dr. Posnick,

I am a former patient of yours that was always alone at the hospital with no parents. I was the little girl with a massive hemangioma on the left side of my face. You fixed it with surgery and tissue expanders. I never forgot you after all these years and am still thankful for your help in the 1980s. I have been married for 12 years now, own a construction business, and have 4 children. In honor of my memories of you and how you changed my life by fixing my face, I named my son Jeffrey and told him the whole story and the doctor I named him after.

Sincerely,
Laura Wakeg

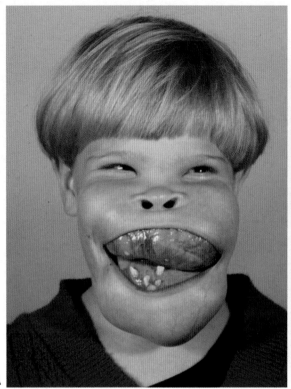

A

5 yr old girl

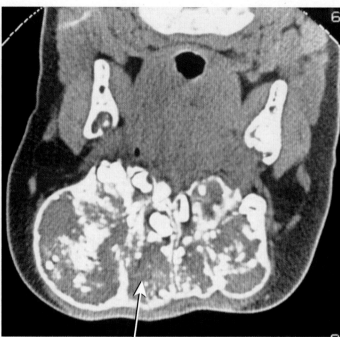

extensive fibrous dysplasia of bone

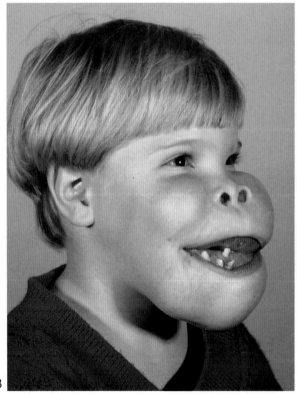

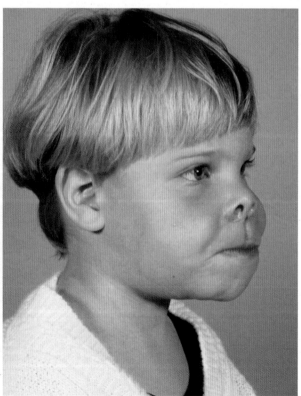

B

before & after tumor resection & reconstruction

• **Figure 5.1** A 5-year-old girl with polyostotic fibrous dysplasia with massive involvement of the maxilla and mandible bilaterally. An asymmetric swelling of the mandible (left greater than right) was first recognized when the child was 18 months old; it rapidly enlarged, and maxillary involvement became evident with deterioration of breathing, chewing, speech, and swallowing. Pathologic fractures were sustained in the extremities as a result of systemic involvement of fibrous dysplasia. **A,** Facial and computed tomography (CT) scan views before facial surgery. **B,** Oblique facial views before and after reconstruction confirming improved lip closure.

Continued

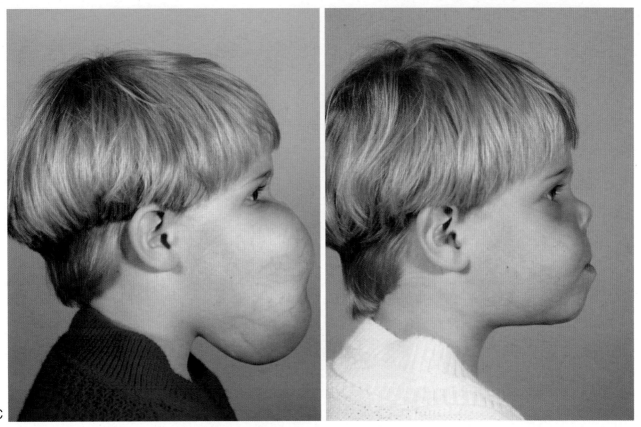

C

before & after tumor resection & reconstruction

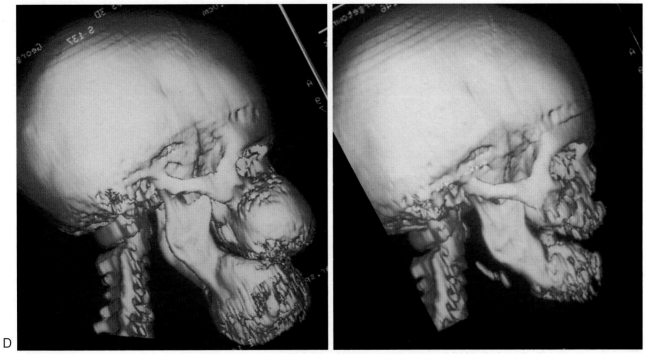

D

CT scan views before & after tumor resection & reconstruction

Figure 5.1, cont'd C, Profile views before and after reconstruction confirming improved lip closure. **D,** CT views before and after debulking procedure. (A–D) From Posnick JC, Hughes CA, Milmoe G, et al. Polyostotic fibrous dysplasia: An unusual presentation in childhood. *J Oral Maxillofac Surg*. 1996;54:1458.

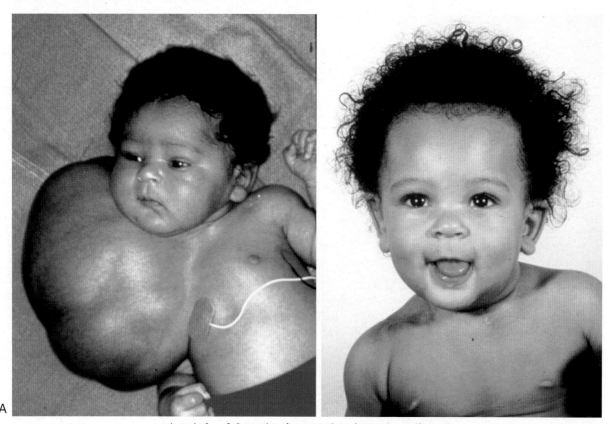

A

newborn before & 6 months after resection of vascular malformation

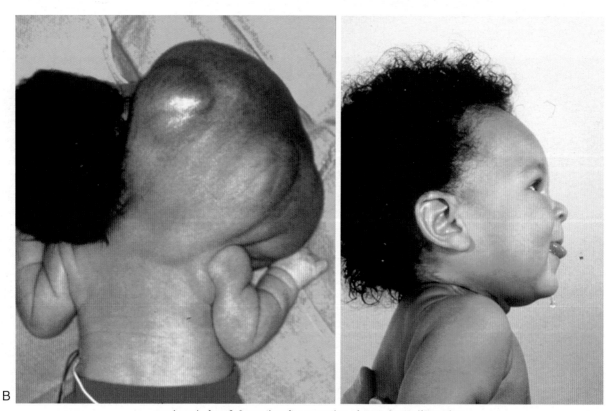

B

newborn before & 6 months after resection of vascular malformation

• **Figure 5.2** A newborn child with a massive low-flow mixed (lymphatic-venous) vascular malformation involving the right side of the face, neck, chest wall, upper arm, and upper back. The malformation was recognized through ultrasonic evaluation during fetal development, and the child was delivered by Cesarean section with a good airway. At 6 weeks of age he underwent an urgent surgical debulking procedure. He is shown before and 6 months after a single-stage excision and reconstruction and then at 5 years of age without recurrence. He has good cranial nerve and brachial plexus function. Portions of the sternocleidomastoid, trapezius, and platysma muscles were sacrificed in the process. **A,** Frontal views before and at 7 months of age, after resection. **B,** Posterior views before and at 7 months of age, after resection.

Continued

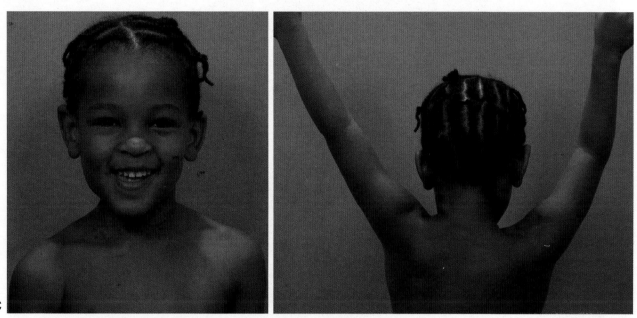

5 yrs of age after tumor resection without recurrence

Figure 5.2, cont'd C, Frontal and posterior views at 5 years of age without recurrence. (A–C) From Posnick JC. Hemangiomas and vascular malformations of the head and neck: Evaluation and management. *Craniofacial and Maxillofacial Surgery in Children and Young Adults* (JC Posnick, ed.). Philadelphia: W.B. Saunders Co. Ch. 26, Fig. 26-11; 2000.

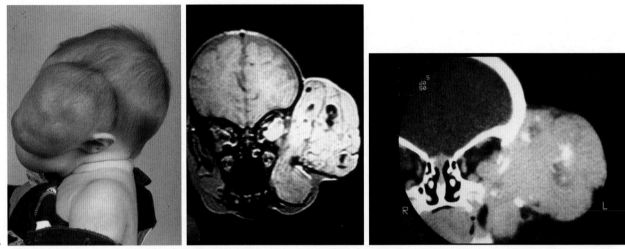

6 mo. old girl with low flow mixed vascular malformation

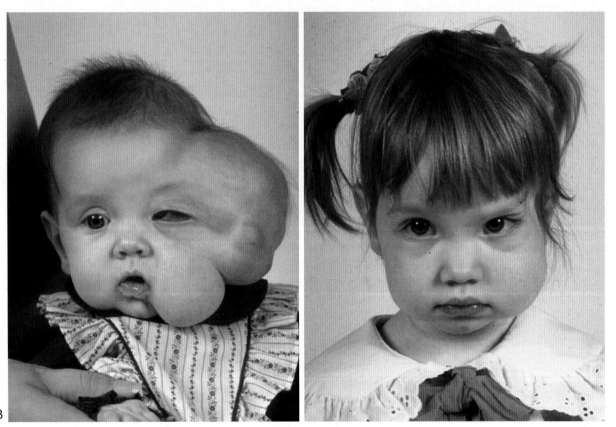

before & 1 yr after resection of vascular malformation

• **Figure 5.3** A child born with a massive low-flow (venous) vascular malformation involving the left side of the face underwent removal at 6 months of age. She is shown before and 1 year after surgical debulking, with facial nerve preservation
carried out through a preauricular and coronal (scalp) incision. **A,** Preoperative oblique facial and magnetic resonance imaging (MRI) and CT scan views through the craniofacial region demonstrating vascular malformation of the left face and orbit.
B, Frontal views before and after debulking and reconstruction.

Continued

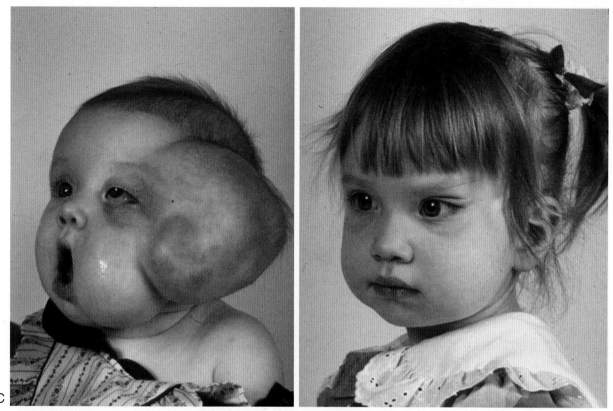

before & 1 yr after resection of vascular malformation

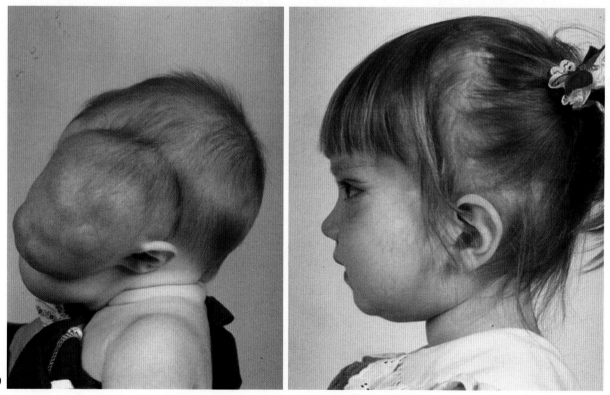

before & 1 year after resection of vascular malformation

Figure 5.3, cont'd C, Oblique views before and after reconstruction. **D,** Profile views before and after reconstruction.

Continued

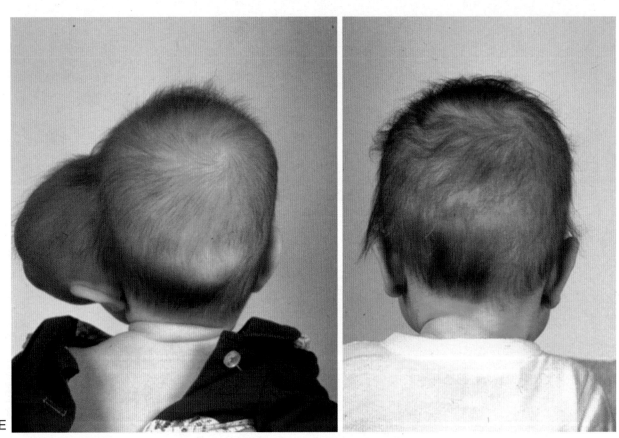

before & 1 year after resection of vascular malformation

Figure 5.3, cont'd E, Posterior views before and after reconstruction. (A–E From Posnick JC. Hemangiomas and vascular malformations of the head and neck: Evaluation and management. *Craniofacial and Maxillofacial Surgery in Children and Young Adults* (JC Posnick, ed.). Philadelphia: W.B. Saunders Co. Ch. 26, pp. 565–596; 2000.

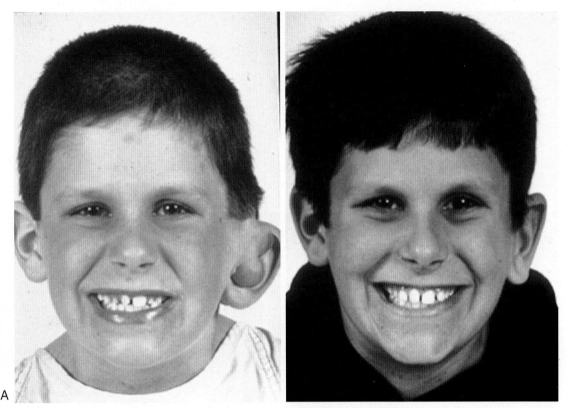

before & 1 year after debulking of vascular malformation

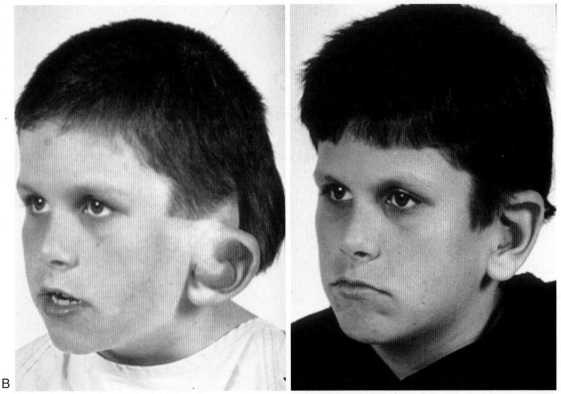

before & 1 year after debulking of vascular malformation

• **Figure 5.4** A 10-year-old boy with a low-flow (venous) vascular malformation involving the left auricular, post-auricular, and occipito-parietal regions. He is shown before and 1 year after undergoing surgical debulking. **A,** Frontal view before and after reconstruction. **B,** Oblique facial view before and after reconstruction.

Continued

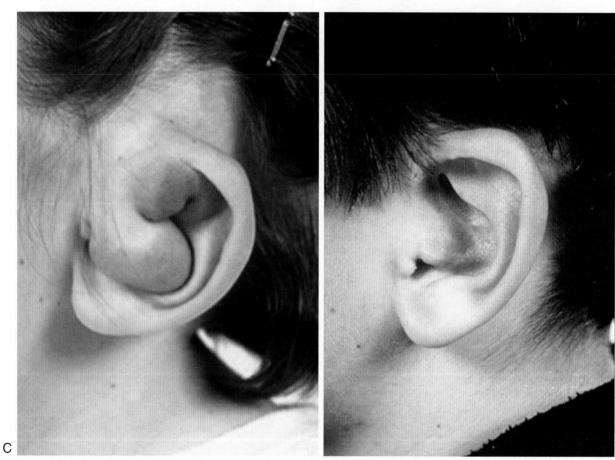

before & 1 year after debulking of vascular malformation

Figure 5.4, cont'd C, Close-up of ear before and after reconstruction. (A–C) From Posnick JC. Hemangiomas and vascular malformations of the head and neck: Evaluation and management. *Craniofacial and Maxillofacial Surgery in Children and Young Adults* (JC Posnick, ed.). Philadelphia: W.B. Saunders Co. Ch. 26, pp. 583–584; 2000.

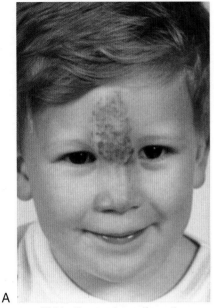

A   Child with vascular malformation
of forehead

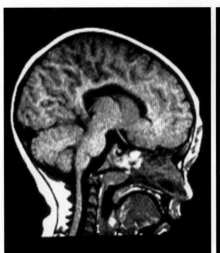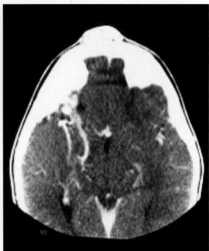

B   MRI confirms only extra-cranial involvement

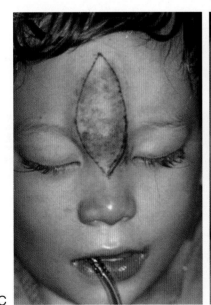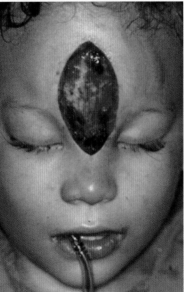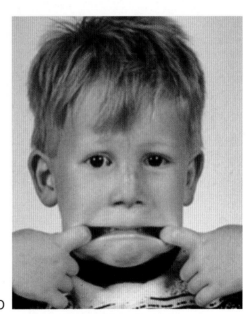

C   vertical midline excision – flap advancement – direct closure   D   several months later

• **Figure 5.5** A 3-year-old boy born with a low-flow (venous) vascular malformation of the central forehead. He is shown before and after undergoing a direct vertical midline excision and flap advancement closure. **A,** Frontal view before surgery. **B,** Preoperative mid-sagittal MRI through the cranium and scalp and coronal CT slice through the mid-forehead, both demonstrating an extracranial vascular malformation. **C,** Intraoperative view demonstrating planned excision, defect after excision just prior to flap advancement and primary wound closure. **D,** Frontal view after reconstruction. (A–D) From Posnick JC. Hemangiomas and vascular malformations of the head and neck: Evaluation and management. *Craniofacial and Maxillofacial Surgery in Children and Young Adults* (JC Posnick, ed.). Philadelphia: W.B. Saunders Co. Ch. 26, p. 580; 2000.

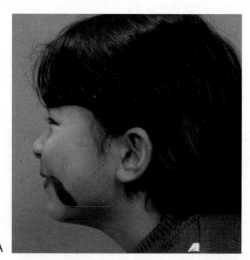

4 yr old with congenital nevi

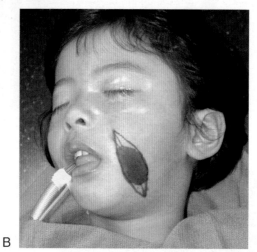

Planned full thickness excision

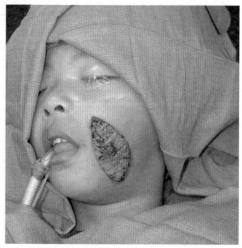

Prior to flap undermining & advancement

• **Figure 5.6** A 4-year-old child with congenital nevi (pigmented lesion) located in the left anterior cheek of the face region. The lesion is not only unsightly but has potential for malignant transformation over a lifetime. The only available treatment is surgical excision with histologic examination to confirm the lesion's character. The lesion was excised full thickness with immediate local flap reconstruction. **A–C,** Profile facial and intraoperative views demonstrating excision of nevi prior to flap advancement for primary closure.

Continued

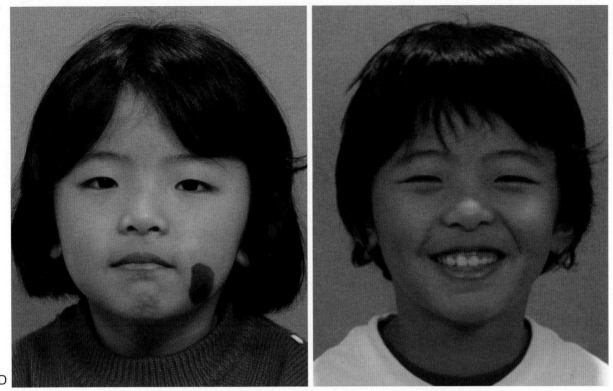

before & after removal of congenital nevi with flap advancement closure

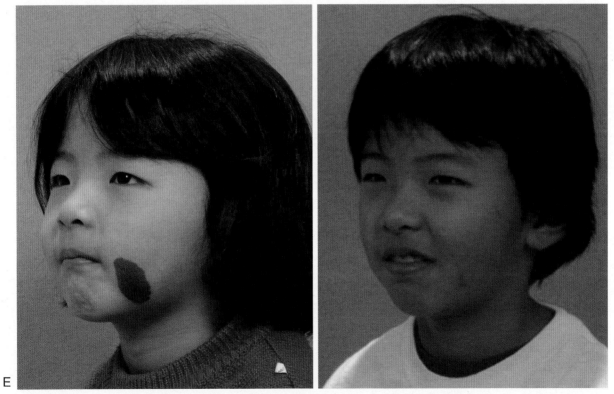

before & after removal of congenital nevi with flap advancement closure

Figure 5.6, cont'd D, Frontal facial views before and after excision and reconstruction. **E**, Oblique facial views before and after excision reconstruction.

References

1. Cohen Jr MM. Vascular update: morphogenesis, tumors, malformations, and molecular dimensions. *Am J Med Genet.* 2006;140A:2013–2038.

2. Abramowicz S, Goldwaser BR, Troulis MJ, Padwa BL, Kaban LB. Primary jaw tumors in children. *J Oral Maxillofac Surg.* 2013;71:47–52.

3. Mulliken JB, Glowacki J. Hemangiomas and vascular malformations in infants and children: a classification based on endothelial characteristics. *Plast Reconstr Surg.* 1982;69:412–422.

4. Posnick JC, Al-Qattan MM, Zuker RM. Large vascular malformation of the face undergoing resection with facial nerve preservation in infancy. *Ann Plast Surg.* 1993;30(1):67–70.

5. Posnick JC. Hereditary, developmental and environmental influences in the formation of dentofacial deformities. In: Posnick JC, ed., Kinard B, assoc. ed. *Orthognathic Surgery: Principles and Practice.* 2nd ed. St. Louis: Elsevier; 2022. ch. 4.

6

Otoplasty for Setback of Protruding Ears

JEFFREY C. POSNICK, DMD, MD

Protruding ears in humans represents a failure in the embryologic development of the underlying cartilage framework. Variations in the cartilage framework are typically seen in two specific locations and cause common patterns of external ear deformity. The first common embryologic error in cartilage development is in the ear fold (i.e., called the antihelical fold). When the antihelical fold is partially or completely absent, the ear will excessively protrude (see Fig. 6.1). The second common malformation of the external ear cartilage framework occurs in the depth of the conchal bowl. When the ear is viewed from the front, if the conchal bowl is excessively deep the ear protrudes too far from the side of the head (see Fig. 6.2).

It was in the 1880s when an American surgeon first described a successful ear setback operation.[1] In his 1910 publication Dr. William Luckett explained the rationale for such an operation.[2] He stated: "It is not enough [for a clinician] to tell a mother of a child that repeatedly returns home from school crying because he has been called donkey ears [to not be concerned] – for such advice will not be accepted [by the child] as the constant harassing by his classmates frequently is the cause of so much distress as to produce a very bad mental condition in the child as well as the parents."

Today, an otoplasty procedure is carried out through an inconspicuous incision made in the skin behind each ear. The incision provides the surgeon access to alter the ear cartilage framework. The ear is reconstructed through a combination of cartilage excision to decrease the depth of the conchal bowl and the placement of sutures to improve the antihelical fold (see Figs. 6.1–6.2). If successfully executed, this will create ideal curvatures of the external ears which optimizes facial appearance (see Figs. 6.3–6.6).[3,4]

An ear setback otoplasty procedure can be safely and definitively performed between 3 and 5 years of age, once ear growth is mature. This is also at an age before negative consequences from the ear deformities on the child's self-esteem will have occurred. As a result of the otoplasty procedure, the ears should no longer draw negative attention from the casual observer at conversational distance. In fact, patient-based quality of life health surveys confirm the positive effects of surgery carried out to correct protruding ears on the child's social interactions, self-esteem, and school performance.[5]

Today, an otoplasty procedure for a child with "outstanding" ears is accomplished under general anesthesia, on an outpatient basis. The compressive ear bandage is removed after 5 days. By 2 weeks after surgery, few limitations remain.[6] Once successful healing has occurred the positive results are expected to last a lifetime. Unfortunately, many families remain unaware that this procedure can be safely and predictably accomplished with important benefits for their child.

Letter from a Past Patient

Hi Dr. Posnick,

I'm now finishing college and want you to know how much I appreciate what you did for me. You set my ears back when I was in high school. I just wish I would have had the surgery sooner. Before the surgery I would always be worried, not knowing when someone would make fun of me. Sometimes I would just avoid being with people altogether. Now I don't even think about it. Even the barber can't see the scars!

Thanks,
Jack Tanner

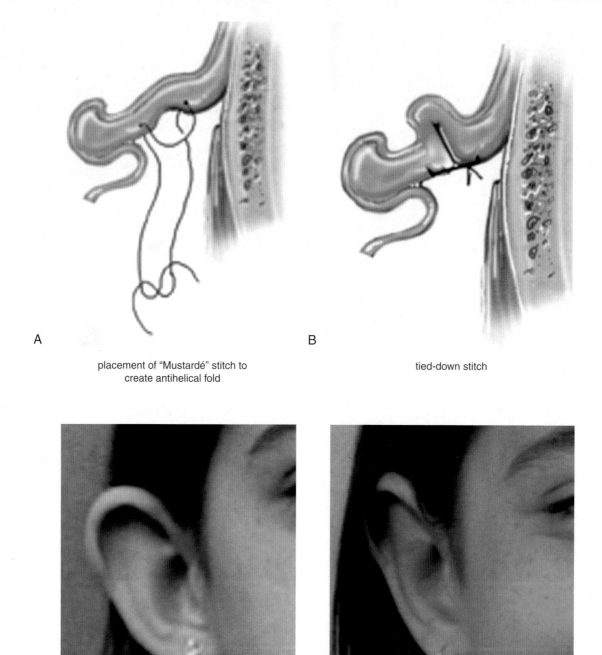

A

placement of "Mustardé" stitch to
create antihelical fold

B

tied-down stitch

C

D

before & after creation of antihelical fold

• **Figure 6.1** Antihelical fold correction. **A,** Illustration of the placement of a "Mustardé" stitch before tie-down (cross-section view). **B,** Illustration of a tied-down "Mustardé" stitch (cross-section view). **C and D,** A child with an absent antihelical fold before and after surgical creation/correction. (A–C) From Posnick, JC. Aesthetic alteration of the prominent ears: Evaluation and surgery. *Orthognathic Surgery: Principles and Practice*, 2nd ed. (JC Posnick, ed., B Kinard, assoc. ed.). St. Louis: Elsevier. Ch. 39, Fig. 39-6, p. 2101; 2022.

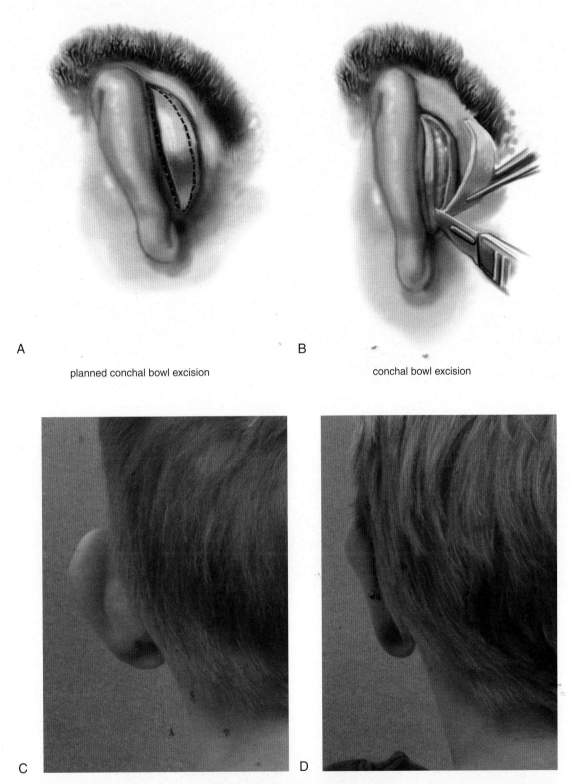

A

planned conchal bowl excision

B

conchal bowl excision

C

D

before & after deep conchal bowl excision

• **Figure 6.2** Deep conchal bowl correction. **A,** Illustration of postauricular approach for access and then for the excision of the ellipse of the conchal wall. **B,** Illustration of scalpel excision of the cartilage ellipse. **C and D,** A child with a deep conchal bowl before and after surgical correction. (A–D) From Posnick JC. Aesthetic alteration of the prominent ears: Evaluation and surgery. *Orthognathic Surgery: Principles and Practice*, 2nd ed. (JC Posnick, ed., B Kinard, assoc. ed.). St. Louis: Elsevier. Ch. 39, Fig. 39-8, p. 2102; 2022.

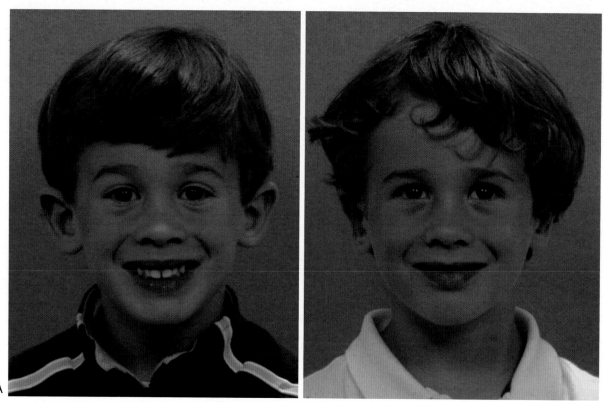

5 yr old before & after ear setback surgery

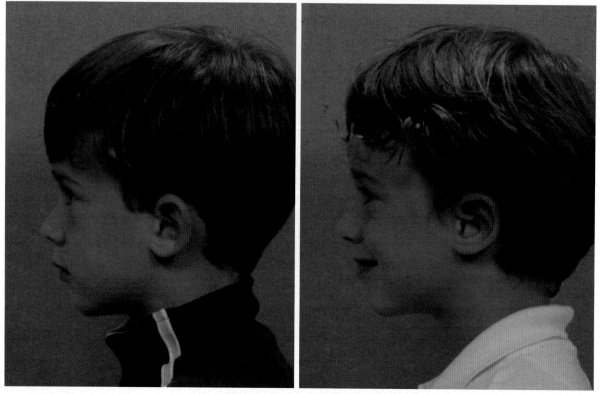

5 yr old before & after ear setback surgery

• **Figure 6.3** A 5-year-old boy with asymmetric prominent and cupped ears characterized by conchal (bowl) hypertrophy, deficient scaphal (antihelical) folding, and a prominent earlobe. He underwent conchal wall resection; conchal rotation and stabilization (conchal–mastoid sutures); improvement of the antihelical folding (Mustardé sutures); and earlobe setback. **A,** Frontal views before and after reconstruction. **B,** Profile views before and after reconstruction.

Continued

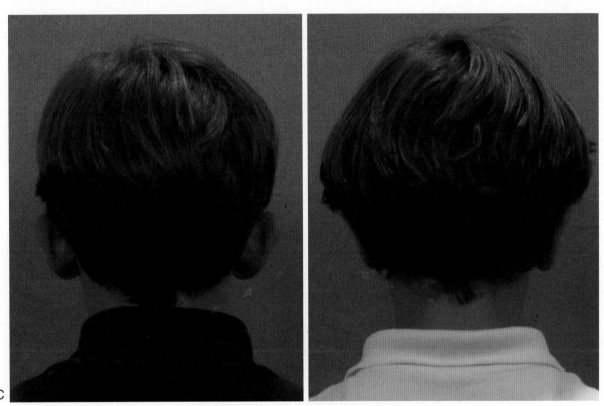

C

5 yr old before & after ear setback surgery

Figure 6.3, cont'd **C,** Posterior facial views before and after reconstruction. (A–C) From Posnick JC. Aesthetic alteration of the prominent ears: Evaluation and surgery. *Orthognathic Surgery: Principles and Practice*, 2nd ed. (JC Posnick, ed., B Kinard, assoc. ed.). St. Louis: Elsevier. Ch. 39, Fig. 39-14, pp. 2111–2112; 2022.

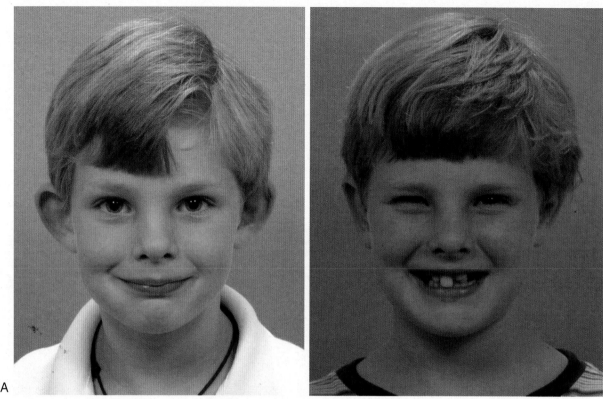

A

5 yr old before & after ear setback surgery

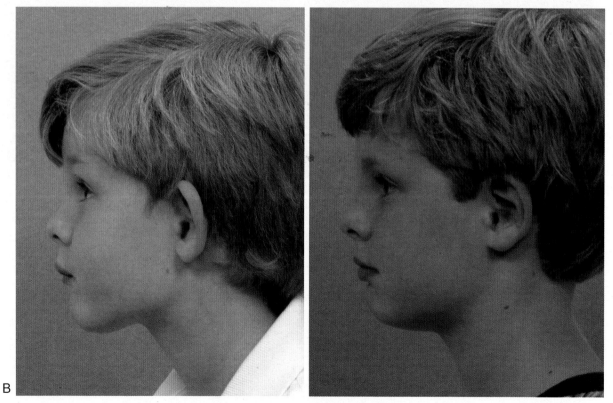

B

5 yr old before & after ear setback surgery

• **Figure 6.4** A 5-year-old boy with small and prominent ears characterized by the absence of scaphal (antihelical) folding and deep conchal (bowl) hypertrophy. He underwent elliptical conchal wall resection; conchal rotation and stabilization (conchal–mastoid sutures); and the creation of antihelical folds (Mustardé sutures). **A,** Frontal views before and after reconstruction. **B,** Profile views before and after reconstruction.

Continued

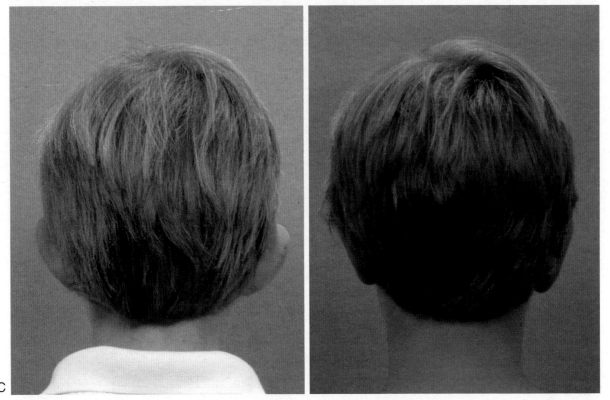

5 yr old before & after ear setback surgery

Figure 6.4, cont'd C, Posterior views before and after reconstruction. (A–C) From Posnick JC. Aesthetic alteration of the prominent ears: Evaluation and surgery. *Orthognathic Surgery: Principles and Practice*, 2nd ed. (JC Posnick, ed., B Kinard, assoc. ed.). St. Louis: Elsevier. Ch. 39, Fig. 39-16, pp. 2115–2116; 2022.

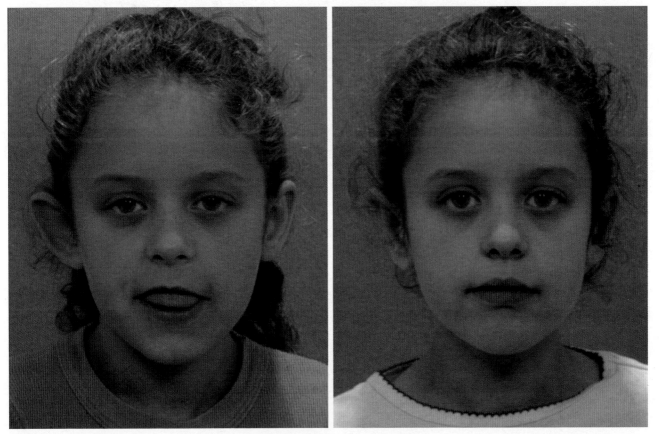

9 yr old before & after ear setback surgery

• **Figure 6.5** A 9-year-old girl with a unilateral prominent ear characterized by the absence of antihelical folding and deep conchal bowl hypertrophy. She underwent a unilateral otoplasty requiring conchal rotation and setback (conchal–mastoid sutures) and the creation of antihelical folding (Mustardé sutures). She is shown before and after unilateral (right side) ear setback surgery. From Posnick JC. Aesthetic alteration of the prominent ears: Evaluation and surgery. *Orthognathic Surgery: Principles and Practice*, 2nd ed. (JC Posnick, ed., B Kinard, assoc. ed.). St. Louis: Elsevier. Ch. 39, Fig. 39-21, p. 2126; 2022.

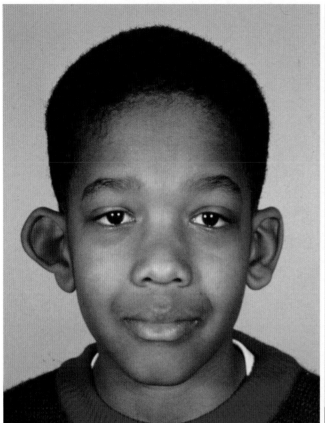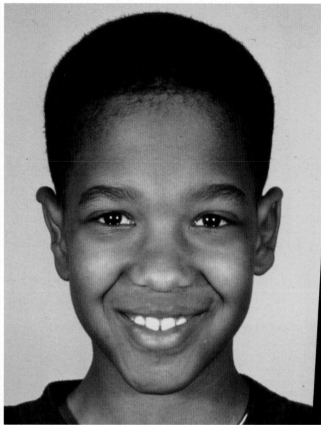

9 yr old before & after ear setback surgery

• **Figure 6.6** A 9-year-old boy with malformed and asymmetric external ears who underwent reconstruction. The procedure included asymmetric elliptical conchal wall resection; conchal rotation and stabilization (conchal–mastoid and superior helix–mastoid sutures); the creation of the antihelical fold (Mustardé sutures); and earlobe setback (soft-tissue sutures). He is shown before and after ear setback surgery. From Posnick JC. Aesthetic alteration of the prominent ears: Evaluation and surgery. *Orthognathic Surgery: Principles and Practice*, 2nd ed. (JC Posnick, ed., B Kinard, assoc. ed.). St. Louis: Elsevier. Ch. 39, Fig. 39-22, p. 2127; 2022.

References

1. Ely E. An operation for prominence of the auricles. *Arch Otolaryngol.* 1881;10:97.
2. Luckett WH. A new operation for prominent ears based on the anatomy of the deformity. *Surg Gynecol Obstet.* 1910;10:635.
3. Gibson TW, Davis W. The distortion of autogenous cartilage grafts: its cause and prevention. *Br J Plast Surg.* 1958;10:257.
4. Mustardé JC. The correction of prominent ears by using simple mattress sutures. *Br J Plast Surg.* 1963;16:170.
5. Litschel R, Majoor J, Tasman A-J. Effect of protruding ears on visual fixation time and perception of personality. *JAMA Facial Plast Surg.* 2015;17(3):183–189.
6. Posnick JC. Aesthetic alteration of the prominent ears: evaluation and surgery. In: Posnick JC, ed., Kinard B, assoc. ed. *Orthognathic Surgery: Principles and Practice.* 2nd ed. St. Louis: Elsevier; 2022. ch. 39.

7

Reconstruction of Developmental Jaw Deformities

JEFFREY C. POSNICK, DMD, MD

Developmental jaw deformities are not present at birth but only progress later during childhood and become apparent early in the teenage years. The resulting jaw disharmony causes malocclusion with expected difficulties in the child's chewing ability, speech articulation, and breathing. The facial disproportions will also tend to have negative effects on the teenager's self-esteem. Ideally, these developmental jaw deformities (also called dentofacial deformities), which occur in approximately 5% of teenagers, should be corrected once facial growth is complete and prior to high school graduation. The optimal correction requires a coordinated orthodontic and jaw surgical approach. The procedures carried out typically include the surgical repositioning of the upper jaw, the lower jaw, and the bone in the chin region (see Fig. 7.1).

The first reported surgical correction of a developmental jaw deformity was carried out in St. Louis, Missouri in 1897. The lower jaw surgery was performed on a 23-year-old medical student. The operation was successfully accomplished by Dr. Vilray P. Blair under ether anesthesia in coordination with orthodontic treatment.[1,2] It was decades later before advanced jaw surgical techniques were innovated by Dr. Hugo Obwegeser in Europe.[3] Obwegeser first presented his work to North America during a three-day invited symposium, including live surgery (June 1966) in Washington, DC, at the Walter Reed Army Hospital. *Time Magazine* was there to document the event and file their report in the July 1, 1966 international edition.[4] The reporter stated: "Last

week, 500 of the most prominent US Oral Surgeons sat on the edge of their chairs at Washington's Walter Reed Army Medical Center, as a respected Swiss practitioner [Obwegeser] described his radical, jaw-splitting procedures for correcting severe malformations."[4] Through experimental studies, Dr. William Bell (Texas surgeon) went on to prove the biologic safety of the Obwegeser procedures, giving surgeons around the world the confidence needed to proceed with jaw reconstruction for their patients.[5] The introduction by Dr. Hans Luhr (German surgeon) of specially designed small metal plates and screws used to internally fixate the jaw bones in their new locations during surgery made these operations more predictable.[6]

Health experts agree that the ultimate determinant of a treatment's success should be heavily judged by the individual's personal satisfaction. The medical literature confirms a high level of patient-rated satisfaction after corrective jaw surgery for the parameters of optimal facial aesthetics (i.e., self-esteem and body image), improved function (i.e., speech articulation, chewing ability, and breathing), and long-term dental health.[7] Today, experienced clinicians are able to safely and effectively complete jaw straightening surgery under general anesthesia followed by an anticipated one- to two-night hospital stay.[8–10] By 5 weeks, the teenager can expect to return to a chewing diet and most sports activities (see Figs. 7.2–7.4). In the future, the proven techniques of jaw reconstruction should become more readily available to all teenagers in need.

Letters from Past Patients

Dear Dr. Posnick,

I want to thank you for completing my jaw surgery when I was a teenager. Over the years since the surgery, I have grown to appreciate improvements in my quality of life. My sleep apnea has gone away! I am no longer dependent on daily naps after work, and I am able to wake up refreshed and go to the gym and start my day early. Previously, this was an impossible feat. It is a testament to just how important sleep is within a person's life. I also have a much better sense of taste and smell as I can breathe better through my nose. All of my teeth now touch when I chew which is great. The surgery has had a positive domino effect throughout my entire life as I also feel better about the way that I look and socialize with others.

Thank you for changing my life.
Kevin Barnes

Dear Dr. Posnick,

I want to thank you and your team for taking such great care of our daughter. You made the difficult and involved surgery seem predictable and feel safe which was very helpful to us as parents. Sarah loves her improved bite, facial appearance, and ability to breathe through her nose. It has given her extra confidence and physical ability in sports.

Sincerest regards,
Cindy and Louis Greene

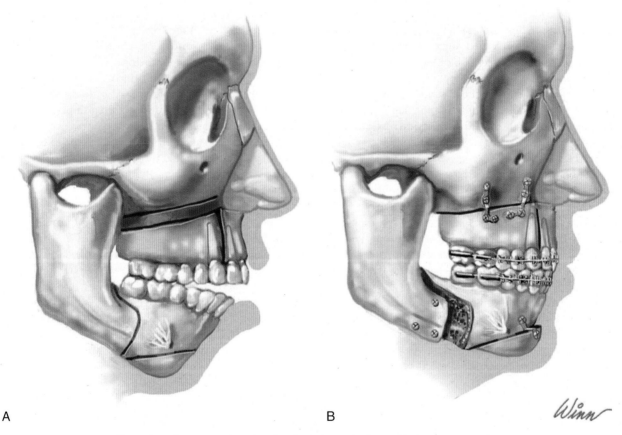

A   B

illustrations demonstrate location of osteotomies typically used for jaw reconstruction

• **Figure 7.1** The illustrations demonstrate a frequent form of developmental jaw disharmony (i.e., long face jaw growth pattern). They also show the location for the osteotomies typically used for jaw reconstruction. The osteotomies are similar to those initially innovated by Obwegeser in the 1960s. They include: maxillary Le Fort I osteotomy; bilateral sagittal (split) ramus osteotomies of the mandible; and an osteotomy of the chin region. The osteotomies are rigidly fixed in place with titanium plates and screws as pioneered by Luhr, also in the 1960s. **A,** Profile view of a long face developmental jaw deformity. The proposed osteotomies are demonstrated. **B,** The standard jaw osteotomies as described have been completed and are shown rigidly fixated in their new locations.

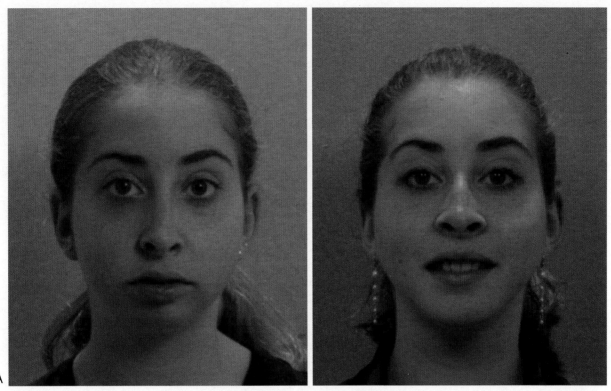

teenager before & after jaw reconstruction

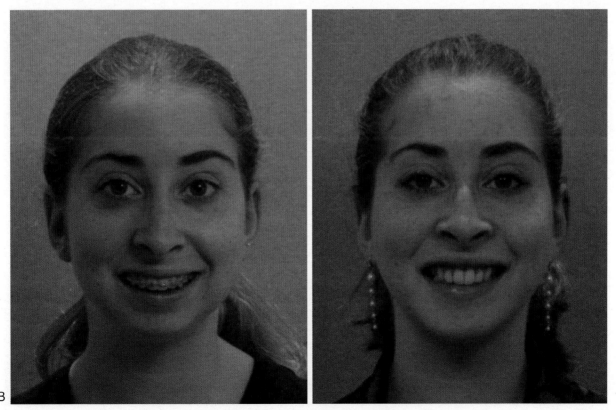

teenager before & after jaw reconstruction

• **Figure 7.2** A 17-year-old girl arrived for a second surgical opinion only after orthodontic treatment was well underway. After referral, this surgeon recommended lower premolar extractions to retract the anterior mandibular teeth in preparation for bimaxillary orthognathic surgery. There was no suggestion of condylar resorption now or in the past. She was also confirmed to have chronic nasal obstruction and mild OSA, which could be simultaneously corrected as part of the jaw reconstruction. The surgery included a maxillary Le Fort I osteotomy in two segments; sagittal (split) ramus osteotomies of the mandible; osseous genioplasty; septoplasty; and inferior turbinate reduction. **A,** Frontal views in repose before and after surgery. **B,** Frontal views with smile before and after surgery.

Continued

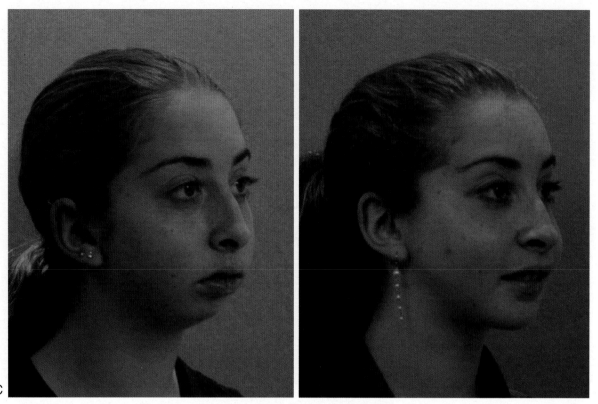

C

teenager before & after jaw reconstruction

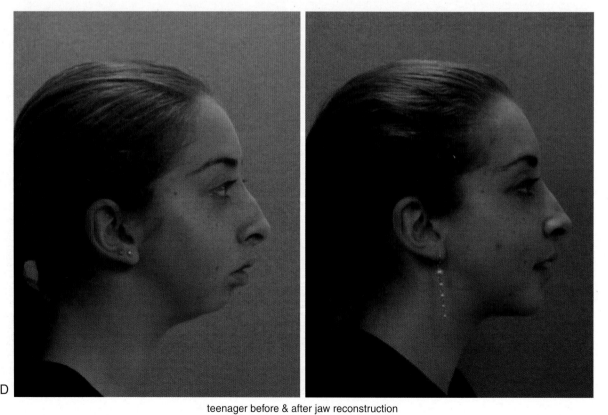

D

teenager before & after jaw reconstruction

Figure 7.2, cont'd C, Oblique facial views before and after surgery. **D,** Profile views before and after surgery.

Continued

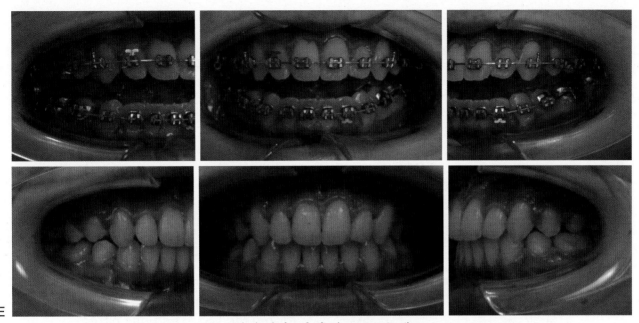

E

occlusion before & after jaw reconstruction

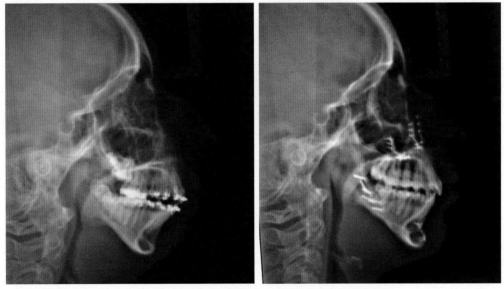

F

cephalometric radiographs before & after jaw reconstruction

Figure 7.2, cont'd **E,** Occlusal views with orthodontics in progress (mandibular premolar extractions) and then after treatment. **F,** Lateral cephalometric radiographs before and after treatment.

Continued

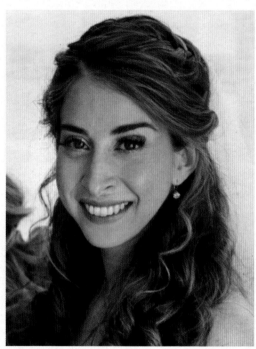

Dr. Posnick,

I wanted to send you my recent wedding photo. The surgery you did for me ten years ago has had a positive impact on my life.

Thank you again!!!

Hannah

G

Figure 7.2, cont'd G, Wedding photograph 10 years after jaw reconstruction. (A–G) From Posnick JC. Primary mandibular deficiency growth patterns. *Orthognathic Surgery: Principles and Practice*, 2nd ed. (JC Posnick, ed., B. Kinard, assoc. ed.). St. Louis: Elsevier. Ch. 19, Fig. 19-14, pp. 765–768; 2022.

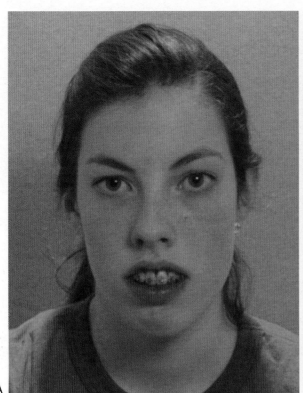
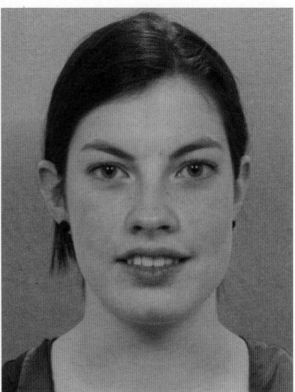

teenager before & after jaw reconstruction

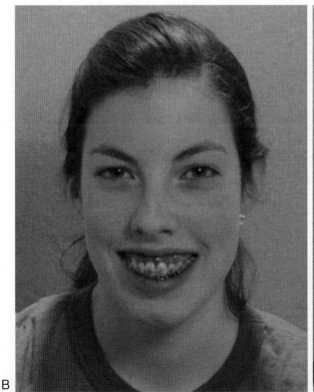
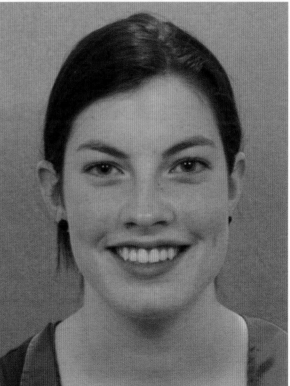

teenager before & after jaw reconstruction

• **Figure 7.3** A 13-year-old girl arrived with her parents for surgical evaluation. She was recognized to have a long face jaw growth pattern. The history and physical examination confirmed lifelong nasal obstruction, lip incompetence, and persistent gingivitis despite good home care. The facial aesthetic concerns included an awareness of a weak chin, a gummy smile, and severe lip strain. Non-extraction orthodontics coordinated with bimaxillary orthognathic and intranasal surgery was agreed to. The simultaneous procedures included Le Fort I osteotomy; sagittal (split) ramus osteotomies of the mandible; osseous genioplasty; septoplasty; inferior turbinate reduction; and nasal floor recontouring. **A,** Frontal views in repose before and after reconstruction. **B,** Frontal views with smile before and after reconstruction.

Continued

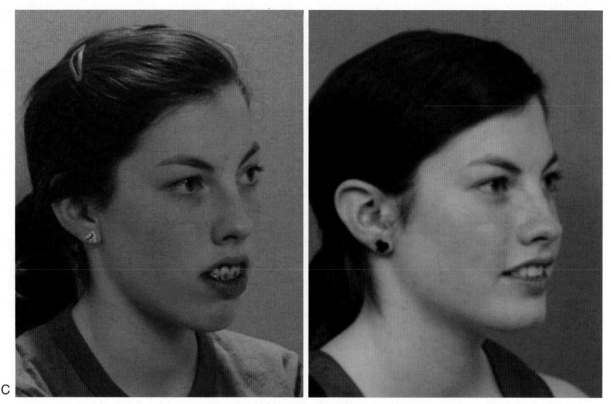

C

teenager before & after jaw reconstruction

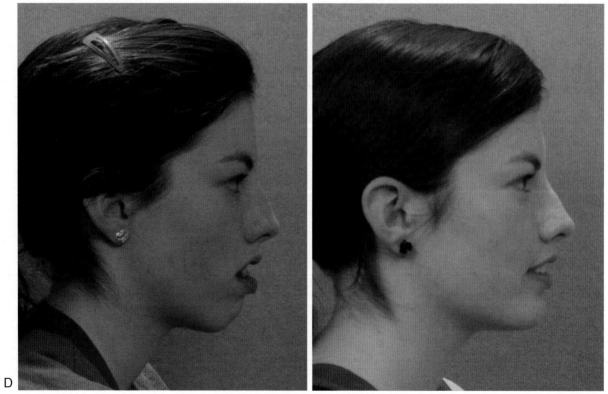

D

teenager before & after jaw reconstruction

Figure 7.3, cont'd C, Oblique facial views before and after reconstruction. D, Profile views before and after reconstruction.

Continued

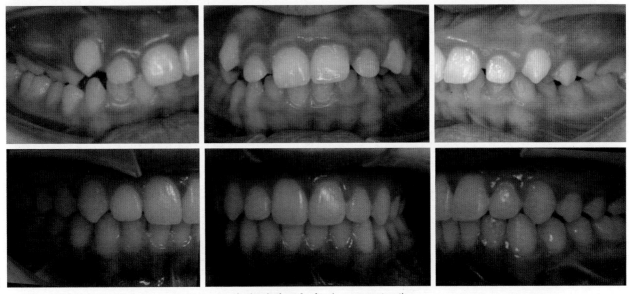

occlusion before & after jaw reconstruction

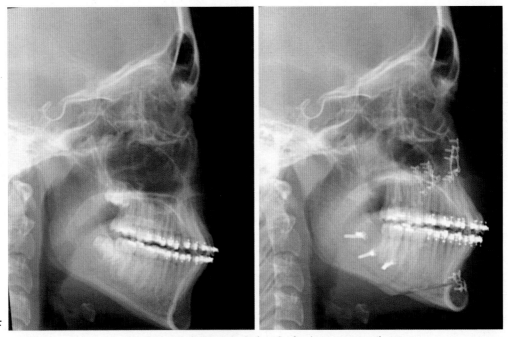

cephalometric radiographs before & after jaw reconstruction

Figure 7.3, cont'd **E,** Occlusal views before treatment and then after completion of treatment. **F,** Lateral cephalometric radiographs before and after surgery. (A–E) From Posnick JC. Long face growth patterns: Maxillary vertical excess with mandibular deformity. *Orthognathic Surgery: Principles and Practice*, 2nd ed. (JC Posnick, ed., B Kinard, assoc. ed.). St. Louis: Elsevier. Ch. 21, Fig. 21-4, pp. 907–910; 2022.

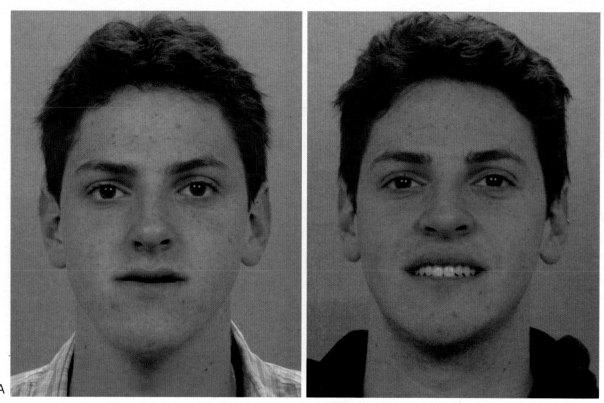

teenager before & after jaw reconstruction

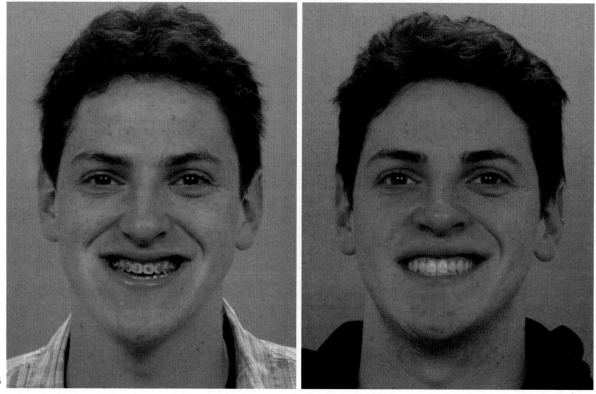

teenager before & after jaw reconstruction

• **Figure 7.4** A 17-year-old boy with a developmental jaw deformity characterized as left-sided hemi-mandibular elongation is shown. This condition affects his chewing, speech articulation, nasal breathing, and facial appearance. He was referred for surgical evaluation at 17 years of age and underwent a coordinated non-extraction orthodontic and a bimaxillary orthognathic approach. The surgery included maxillary Le Fort I osteotomy in two segments; sagittal (split) ramus osteotomies of the mandible; septoplasty; inferior turbinate reduction; and osseous genioplasty. **A,** Frontal views in repose before and then 4 years after reconstruction. **B,** Frontal views with smile before and then 4 years after reconstruction.

Continued

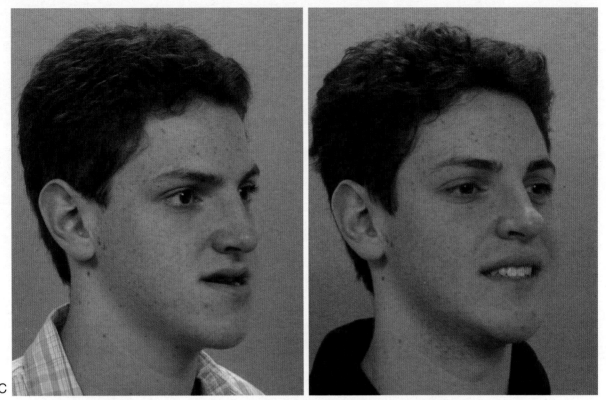

teenager before & after jaw reconstruction

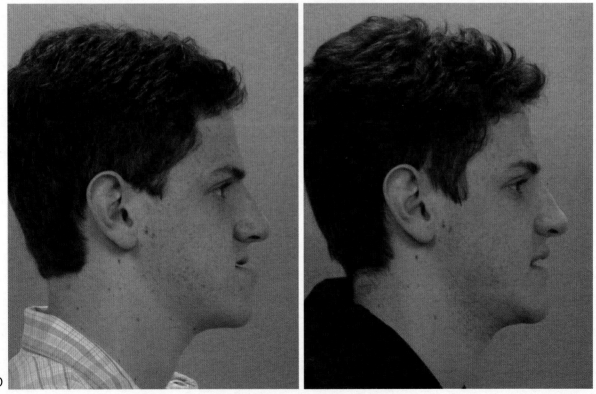

teenager before & after jaw reconstruction

Figure 7.4, cont'd C, Oblique views before and then 4 years after reconstruction. **D,** Profile views before and then 4 years after reconstruction.

Continued

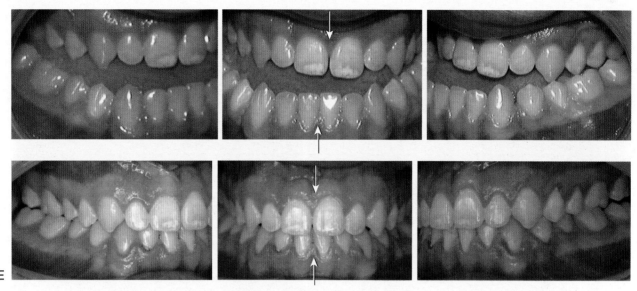

occlusion before & after jaw reconstruction

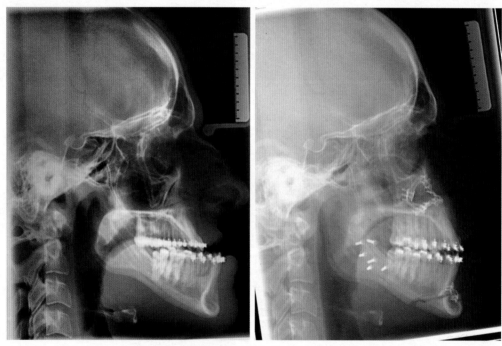

cephalometric radiographs before & after jaw reconstruction

Figure 7.4, cont'd **E,** Occlusal views before retreatment and then 4 years after treatment. **F,** Lateral cephalometric radiographs before and after treatment. (A–F) From Posnick JC, Perez J, Chavda A. Hemi-mandibular elongation: Is the corrected occlusion maintained long-term? Does the mandible continue to grow? *J Oral Maxillofac Surg.* 75:393–395, Fig. 8; 2017.

References

1. Angle EH. Double resection of the lower maxilla. *Dent Cosmos.* 1898;40.
2. Blair VP. Report of a case of double resection for the correction of protrusion of the mandible. *Dent Cosmos.* 1906;48:817–820.
3. Obwegeser HL. Orthognathic surgery and a tale of how three procedures came to be: a letter to the next generations of surgeons. *Clin Plast Surg.* 2007;34:331–355.
4. Oral surgery. a radical new technique. *About Time Mag.* 1966;88:46.
5. Bell WH. Revascularization and bone healing after anterior maxillary osteotomy: a study using adult Rhesus monkeys. *J Oral Surg.* 1969;27:249–255.
6. Luhr HG. Zur stabilen osteosynthese bei unterkiefer-frakturen. *Dtsch Zahnärztl Z.* 1968;23:754.
7. Posnick JC, Wallace J. Complex orthognathic surgery: assessment of patient satisfaction. *J Oral Maxillofac Surg.* 2008;66:934.
8. Posnick JC, Perez J, Chavda A. Hemi-mandibular elongation: is the corrected occlusion maintained long-term? Does the mandible continue to grow? *J Oral Maxillofac Surg.* 2017;75:371–398.
9. Posnick JC, Egolum N, Tremont T. Primary mandibular deficiency dentofacial deformities: occlusion and facial aesthetic surgical outcomes. *J Oral Maxillofac Surg.* 2018;76:2209.e1–2209.e15.
10. Posnick JC, Kinard BE. Orthognathic surgery has a significant positive effect on perceived personality traits and perceived emotional expressions in long face subjects. *J Oral Maxillofac Surg.* 2019;77:408.e1–408.e10.

8
Cleft Lip and Palate Reconstruction

JEFFREY C. POSNICK, DMD, MD

The embryologic development of the face remains somewhat of a mystery despite major scientific advances over the past half century. In fetal life, we all start out with a complete cleft of the upper lip (i.e., the upper lip is in three segments) and with a cleft through the palate (i.e., the palate is also in three segments). By 5–8 weeks of embryologic life, for all but approximately 1 in 1000 newborns, the upper lip and the palate will fuse together in a perfectly normal way. When a child is born with a cleft of the lip and palate (lack of fusion of the facial parts), immediate difficulty with feeding and many other aspects of newborn life are expected. The potential devastating social and economic effects for the family as a whole cannot be overstated and should not be underestimated.[1]

A congenital cleft of the lip and palate has no doubt occurred since early in the development of *Homo sapiens*, and yet even among ancient medical writers congenital clefting gained little attention. Chinese surgeons (229–317 AD) seem to be the first to have reported rudimentary repair of a cleft lip. Ambroise Paré, from France, described the systematic repair of cleft lip in 1568. He did the surgery without the benefit of any type of anesthesia.[3] His technique included "searing" the edges of each side of the cleft with scissors, then bringing the cut edges together, and holding them in place "with needles and string until adequately healed". At that time, an understanding of the cause of a cleft lip was a mystery and open to wide speculation. In 1733, French surgeon Georges De La Faye stated: "The father of a young boy [with a harelip] told me that his wife, who is now dead, had been, in her imagination, frightened by the sight of a lion." The family was convinced that this was the cause of their child's deformity. In another case, a mother of a child with a harelip said that during pregnancy "she had been frightened at the sight of the head of a deer [whose clefted lip resembled that of her child]".[2]

In describing the success of the lip repair operation, De La Faye stated: "The child is now infinitely less deformed than he was before the [cleft lip] operation; one can [now] look at him without a shock." He went on to state: "this is not the only advantage [of the surgery] – he [now] talks distinctly, though a little [air] through the nose [remains] – a [speech] defect he would not have if his palate were [also] entirely closed".[2]

After the advent of ether general anesthesia (1846), surgeons were able to take the necessary time to refine cutting and suturing techniques for congenital lip repair. It was not until the 1960s and 1970s that Ralph Millard (American surgeon) both refined and simplified the standard repair of a cleft lip. Repair of a cleft lip could now be understood and safely executed by a surgeon committed to learning the technique.[4,5] In the 1980s, Harold McComb (Australian surgeon) demonstrated the value of also reconstructing the malformed nasal tip at the same time as the primary cleft lip repair.[6]

Today there are 10 million humans worldwide born with a cleft lip and palate. Some 1.5 million of these children who were otherwise without access to medical care or the financial means have benefited from free primary cleft repair by a "Smile Train" sponsored surgeon and facility (a worldwide charitable organization started in the late 1990s).[7] Presently, cleft lip repair is an operation that can be safely carried out under general anesthesia by a trained surgeon, requiring about 45–60 minutes with the child, who is generally able to immediately return home to the care of their parents (see Figs. 8.1–8.9).[8]

While a meticulous lip repair is an essential first step, a longer journey of staged surgical reconstruction and dental rehabilitation is required. Today, carefully coordinated orthodontic and surgical care should see the teenager graduate from high school no longer required to give special consideration to their original birth malformation (see Chapter 9).

Letter from a Past Patient (see Fig. 8.6)

Dear Dr. Posnick,

We just wanted to take a moment prior to Sarah's surgery to thank you for all your help thus far. Your experience and counsel have done so much to calm our fears and emotions after finding out about our daughter's cleft just a few months ago.

We know that we will have a long way to go but this Friday is certainly a big day for us, especially Sarah when the cleft lip will be repaired. We are confident that she is in good and competent hands and are glad that you will be with us every step along the way.

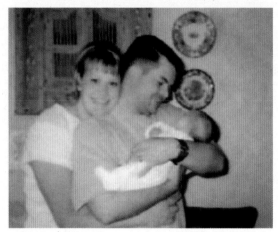

Sincerely yours,
Pamela and James Middlebrook

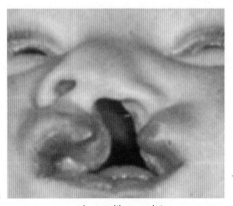

A

newborn with complete
unilateral cleft lip & palate

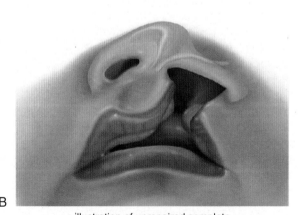

B

illustration of unrepaired complete
unilateral cleft lip & palate

• **Figure 8.1** Illustrations of a typical unilateral cleft lip and palate deformity and the primary repair. **A,** Newborn with unilateral cleft lip and palate (UCLP). **B,** Illustration of typical dysmorphology of newborn with unrepaired UCLP. **C,** Modified "Millard" rotation and advancement flaps used by this surgeon to repair a cleft lip. The incisions are indicated (straight lines) with redundant skin to be excised shown (diagonal lines). **D,** The rotation and advancement skin flaps are elevated. The orbicularis oris muscle is released.

Continued

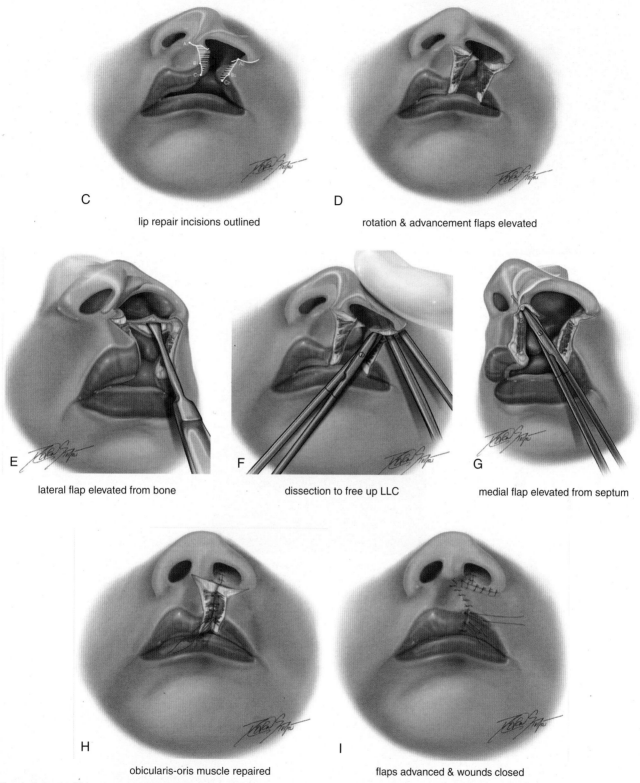

C — lip repair incisions outlined

D — rotation & advancement flaps elevated

E — lateral flap elevated from bone

F — dissection to free up LLC

G — medial flap elevated from septum

H — obicularis-oris muscle repaired

I — flaps advanced & wounds closed

Figure 8.1, cont'd E, The lateral nasal flap is released from the underlying bone and elevated prior to lip repair. **F,** Dissection of the lower lateral cartilage (LLC) from the overlying skin of the nose is completed prior to lip repair. **G,** Along the medial aspect, the nasal soft tissues are released from the anterior nasal spine and septal cartilage. **H,** The released orbicularis oris muscle is sutured across the cleft. **I,** The skin rotation and advancement lip flaps are then approximated and sutured in place to restore the nasal sill and philtral column. (A–I) From Posnick JC. Aesthetic alteration of the nose: Evaluation and surgery. *Orthognathic Surgery: Principles and Practice*, 2nd ed. (JC Posnick, ed., B Kinard, assoc. ed.). St. Louis: Elsevier. Ch. 38, Figs. 38-24, 38-25, 38-26, pp. 2024–2026; 2022.

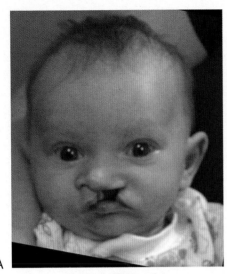

newborn with complete
unilateral cleft lip & palate

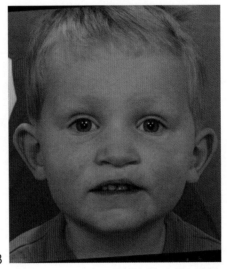

18 mos of age after cleft lip & palate repair

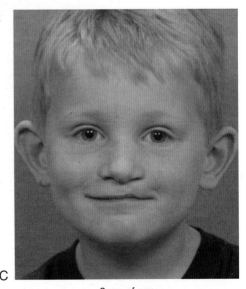

3 yrs of age

• **Figure 8.2** A child born with a UCLP is shown. When he was 3 months old, he underwent primary cleft lip repair and primary nasal reconstruction. When he was 12 months old, he underwent cleft palate repair. He is shown: **A,** as a newborn; **B,** at 18 months of age (6 months after palate repair); and **C,** at 4 years of age. (A–C) From Posnick JC. Aesthetic alteration of the nose: Evaluation and surgery. *Orthognathic Surgery: Principles and Practice*, 2nd ed. (JC Posnick, ed., B Kinard, assoc. ed.). St. Louis: Elsevier. Ch. 38, Fig. 38-27, p. 2027; 2022.

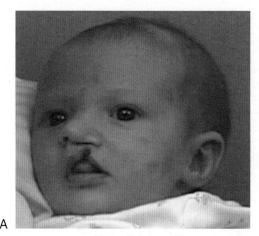

A

newborn with incomplete
unilateral cleft lip & palate

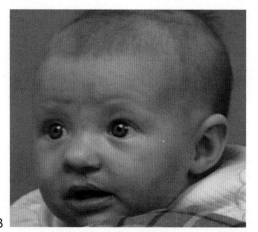

B

1 wk after lip repair

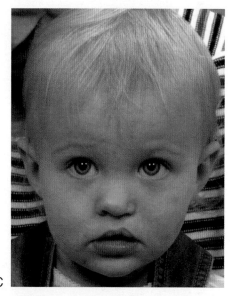

C

1 yr of age

• **Figure 8.3** A child born with an incomplete UCLP is shown. There is nasal deformity and a cleft through the alveolar ridge. At the time of primary cleft lip repair, she also underwent primary nasal reconstruction. This was followed by palate repair when she was 12 months old. She is shown: **A,** as a newborn; **B,** at 3 months of age (1 week after primary lip repair); and **C,** at 1 year of age. (A–C) From Posnick JC. Aesthetic alteration of the nose: Evaluation and surgery. *Orthognathic Surgery: Principles and Practice*, 2nd ed. (JC Posnick, ed., B Kinard, assoc. ed.). St. Louis: Elsevier. Ch. 38, Fig. 38-28, p. 2028; 2022.

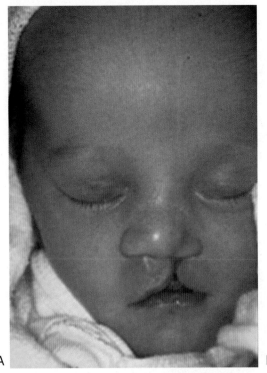

A

newborn with complete unilateral cleft lip & palate

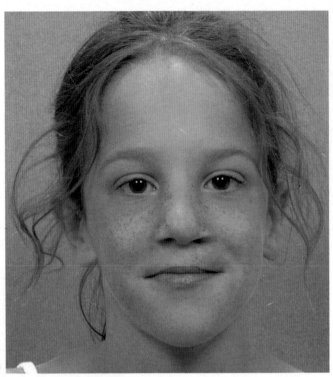

B

8 yrs of age after cleft lip/palate repair

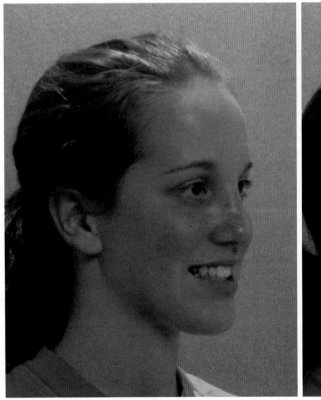

C

15 yrs of age after completion of cleft reconstruction

• **Figure 8.4** A child born with a UCLP is shown. At 3 months of age, she underwent primary cleft lip and cleft nasal reconstruction. When she was 12 months old, she underwent cleft palate repair. She is shown: **A,** as a newborn; **B,** at 8 years of age after primary lip and palate repair; and **C,** at 15 years of age after completion of cleft reconstruction, including need for definitive cleft nasal surgery. (A–C) From Posnick JC. Cleft-orthognathic surgery: The unilateral cleft lip and palate deformity. *Orthognathic Surgery: Principles and Practice*, 2nd ed. (JC Posnick, ed., B Kinard assoc. ed.). St. Louis: Elsevier. Ch. 32, Fig. 32-6, p. 1562–1563; 2022.

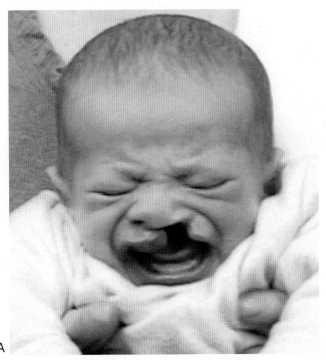

newborn with complete unilateral cleft lip & palate

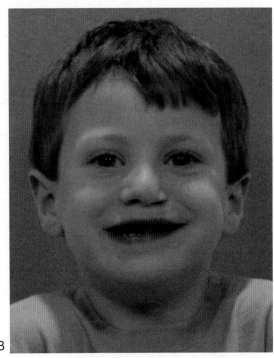

8 yrs of age after cleft lip/palate repair

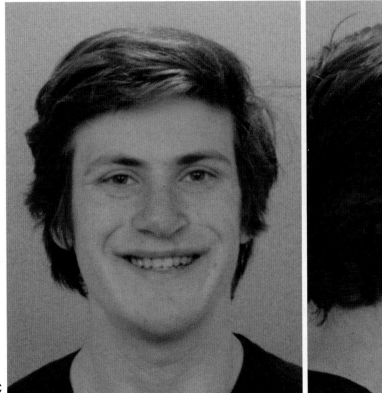

17 yrs of age after completion of cleft reconstruction

• **Figure 8.5** A child born with a UCLP is shown. At 3 months of age, he underwent primary cleft lip repair and cleft nasal reconstruction. When he was 12 months old, he underwent cleft palate repair. He is shown: **A,** as a newborn; **B,** at 8 years of age after primary lip and palate repair just prior to bone graft procedure; and **C,** at 17 years of age after completion of cleft reconstruction including need for cleft jaw and definitive cleft nasal surgery. (A–C) From Posnick JC. Cleft-orthognathic surgery: The unilateral cleft lip and palate deformity. *Orthognathic Surgery: Principles and Practice*, 2nd ed. (JC Posnick, ed., B Kinard, assoc. ed.). St. Louis: Elsevier. Ch. 32, Fig. 32-13, pp. 1599–1603; 2022.

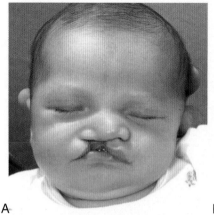
A
newborn with complete unilateral
cleft lip & palate

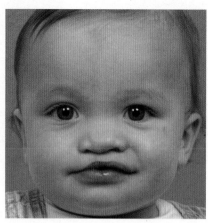
B
1 week after cleft lip repair

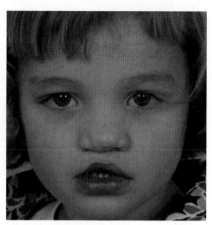
C
7 yrs of age

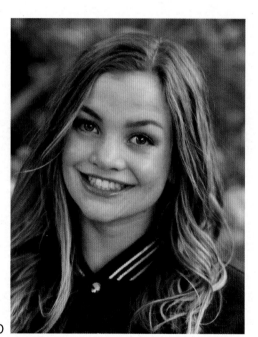
D

Dear Dr. Posnick,

Thank you again for everything that you have done for me and my family over the past 17 years!

Sarah Middlebrook

• **Figure 8.6** A child born with a UCLP is shown. At 3 months of age, she underwent primary cleft lip repair and cleft nasal reconstruction. When she was 12 months old, she underwent cleft palate repair. She is shown: **A,** as a newborn; **B,** at 3 months of age (1 week after primary lip and nose repair); **C,** at 7 years of age just prior to bone graft procedure; and **D,** at high school graduation after completion of cleft reconstruction including need for cleft jaw and definitive cleft nasal surgery. (A–D) From Posnick JC. Aesthetic alteration of the nose: Evaluation and surgery. *Orthognathic Surgery: Principles and Practice*, 2nd ed. (JC Posnick, ed., B Kinard, assoc. ed.). St. Louis: Elsevier. Ch. 38, Fig. 38-29, p. 2029; 2022.

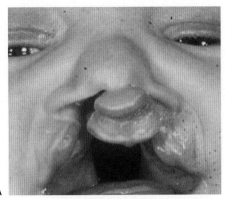

A newborn with complete bilateral
cleft lip & palate

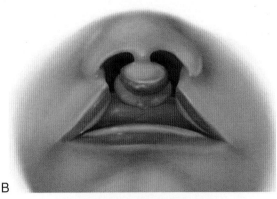

B illustration of unrepaired complete
bilateral cleft lip & palate

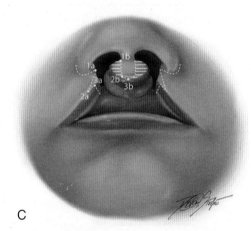

C lip repair incisions outlined

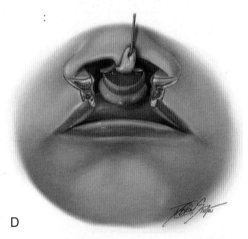

D philtral, rotation & advancement flaps elevated

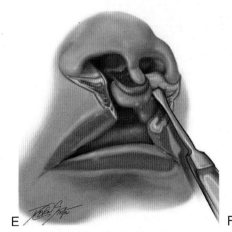

E lateral flap elevated from bone

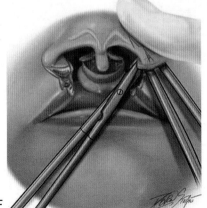

F dissection to free up LLC

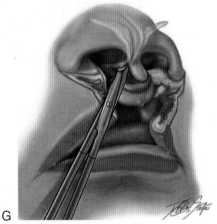

G medial flap elevated from septum

• **Figure 8.7** Illustrations of a typical bilateral cleft lip and palate deformity and the primary repair. **A,** Newborn with bilateral cleft lip and palate (BCLP). **B,** Illustration of typical dysmorphology of newborn with unrepaired BCLP. **C,** The basic bilateral cleft lip reconstruction as carried out by this surgeon. The skin incisions are indicated (dotted lines), with redundant tissue to be excised shown (diagonal lines). **D,** The philtral skin flap has been elevated. The lateral skin flaps including vermilion–mucosa extensions are elevated. The orbicularis oris muscle has been dissected within the lateral flaps. **E and F,** The lateral nasal flaps are released from the underlying bone and elevated. This includes dissection of the lower lateral cartilage (LLC) from the overlying skin of the nose prior to tip repair. **G,** The medial nasal flaps have been dissected and released.

Continued

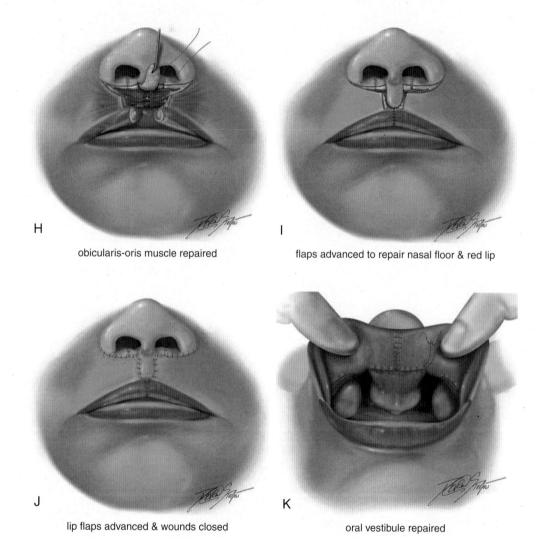

H
obicularis-oris muscle repaired

I
flaps advanced to repair nasal floor & red lip

J
lip flaps advanced & wounds closed

K
oral vestibule repaired

Figure 8.7, cont'd H, The orbicularis oris muscle is approximated across the cleft and sutured. **I,** The vermillion–mucosa extensions of each lateral flap are approximated and sutured in the midline. The anterior aspect of the nasal floor is restored and sutured on each side. **J,** The philtral flap is aligned and sutured at the new vermilion. The lateral skin flaps are advanced, aligned, and sutured to form the nasal sills and the philtral column. **K,** The intraoral mucosa is aligned and sutured to establish a functional vestibule. (A–K) From Posnick JC. Aesthetic alteration of the nose: Evaluation and surgery. *Orthognathic Surgery: Principles and Practice*, 2nd ed. (JC Posnick, ed., B Kinard, assoc. ed.). St. Louis: Elsevier. Ch. 38, Fig. 38-30, Fig. 38-31, Fig. 38-32, pp. 2030–2033; 2022.

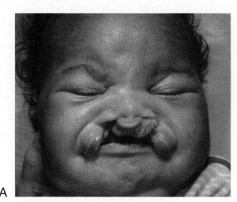

A   newborn with bilateral cleft

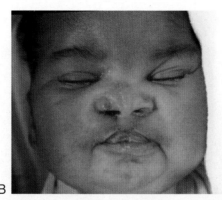

B   1 wk after lip repair

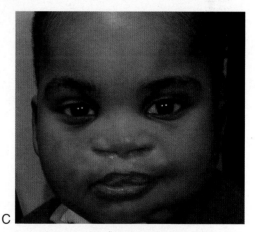

C   2.5 yrs of age after palate repair

• **Figure 8.8** A child born with a complete BCLP, tracheomalacia, and other congenital anomalies is shown. At the time of primary cleft lip repair, he also underwent primary nasal reconstruction. He is shown: **A,** soon after birth and **B,** at 3 months of age, just 1 week after primary cleft lip and nasal reconstruction. **C,** He is next shown at 2.5 years of age having also undergone cleft palate repair. (A–C) From Posnick JC. Aesthetic alteration of the nose: Evaluation and surgery. *Orthognathic Surgery: Principles and Practice*, 2nd ed. (JC Posnick, ed., B Kinard, assoc. ed.). St. Louis: Elsevier. Ch. 38, Fig. 38-33, p. 2034; 2022.

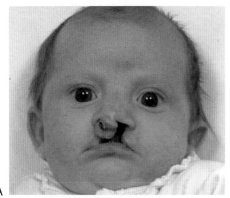

A　newborn with complete bilateral cleft lip & palate

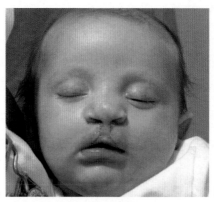

B　1 week after cleft lip repair

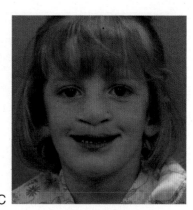

C　7 yrs of age

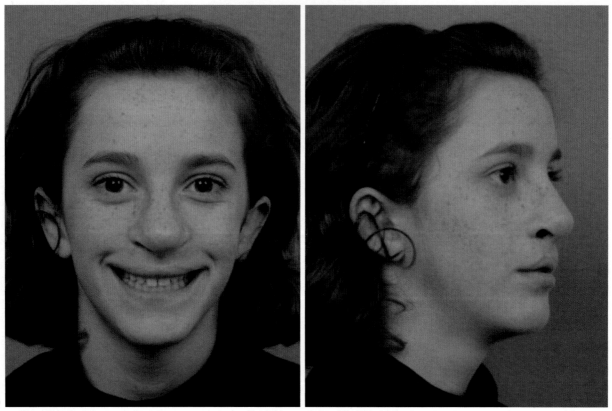

D　15 yrs of age after completion of cleft jaw & nasal reconstruction

• **Figure 8.9** A child born with a complete BCLP is shown. At 3 months of age, she underwent primary cleft lip and cleft nasal reconstruction. When she was 12 months old, she underwent cleft palate repair. She is shown: **A,** as a newborn; **B,** at 1 week after primary cleft lip repair; **C,** at 7 years of age after primary lip and palate repair just prior to bone graft procedure; and **D,** at 15 years of age after completion of reconstruction which included cleft jaw and definitive nasal surgery as a teenager.

Continued

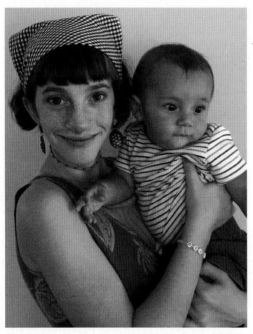

Dear Dr. Posnick,

My dearest plastic surgeon and friend! I am now studying art at college and working as a caregiver for special needs children. I think of you during every milestone in my life and thank you for the big and small acts of love you have shown me.

Eleanor

E

Figure 8.9, cont'd E, During college years. From Posnick JC. Cleft-orthognathic surgery: The bilateral cleft lip and palate deformity. *Orthognathic Surgery: Principles and Practice*, 2nd ed. (JC Posnick ed., B Kinard, assoc. ed.). St. Louis: Elsevier. Ch. 33, Fig. 33-7, pp. 1714–1719; 2022.

References

1. Shaw WC, Brattström V, Mølsted K, Prahl-Andersen B, Roberts CT, Semb G. The Eurocleft study: intercenter study of treatment outcome in patients with complete cleft lip and palate. Part 5: discussion and conclusions. *Cleft Palate Craniofac J*. 2005;42:93.
2. De La Faye G. Observations on the cleft lip. *Memoires de l'Academie Royale de Chirurgie*. 1743;1:605.
3. Paré A. *Les Oeuvres de M. Ambroise Paré*. Paris: G. Bueon; 1575.
4. Millard DR. *Cleft Craft: The Evolution of its Surgery. I. The Unilateral Deformity*. Boston: Little, Brown; 1976.
5. Millard DR. *Cleft Craft: The Evolution of its Surgery. II. Bilateral and Rare Deformities*. Boston: Little, Brown; 1978.
6. McComb H. Primary correction of unilateral cleft lip nasal deformity: a 10-year review. *Plast Reconstr Surg*. 1985;75:791–797.
7. Smile Train. Available at: https://www.smiletrain.org. Accessed July 22, 2020.
8. Posnick JC. Aesthetic alteration of the nose: evaluation and surgery. In: Posnick JC, ed., Kinard B, assoc. ed. *Orthognathic Surgery: Principles and Practice*. 2nd ed. St. Louis: Elsevier; 2022. ch. 38.

9

Cleft Jaw and Cleft Nasal Reconstruction

JEFFREY C. POSNICK, DMD, MD

A congenital cleft of the lip and palate is one of the more common human birth malformations. It is estimated that there are 500,000 citizens in the United States and 10 million people worldwide with cleft lip and palate (see Chapter 8).

The surgical repair of a cleft palate is most frequently carried out before 1 year of age. The timing and rationale for this surgery is to ensure an intact palate for the child to successfully formulate correct and intelligible speech.[1] Unfortunately, repairing the palate at this young age (i.e., prior to 1 year of life) results in scar tissue which frequently inhibits normal growth of the upper jaw (i.e., cleft maxillary hypoplasia) and also causes secondary deformities of adjacent structures (i.e., the lower jaw and nose). By middle school, and then as the jaws complete growth through the early high school years, a severe facial deformity and malocclusion will frequently have occurred.[2] In this circumstance, the negative effects of the cleft jaw deformity on the child's breathing, speech articulation, chewing ability, and self-esteem are unavoidable and persist unless successful reconstruction and coordinated orthodontic treatment is accomplished. The added psychosocial burden for the teenager and the family that is caused by the secondary cleft jaw and nasal deformities over and above the original congenital condition can be daunting.

The procedures for cleft jaw reconstruction are similar but more intricate than those described in Chapter 7 (see Fig. 7.1) for the more routine developmental dentofacial deformities. Safe and effective surgical techniques to correct the secondary jaw and nasal deformities in the teenager with a cleft are known and should be carried out prior to graduation from high school. Unfortunately, the clinical expertise to do so is not yet widely available and accessible to all families in need.[3–5]

The surgery is accomplished under general anesthesia followed by a one- to two-night hospital stay. By 5 weeks after normal expected jaw surgery healing the teenager will restart a chewing diet and return to most sports activities. As early as 6 months after successful jaw surgery, outpatient definitive cleft rhinoplasty with use of a cartilage graft can be carried out to complete the teenager's reconstruction (see Figs. 9.1–9.3).[6–8]

I speak for all professionals caring for children born with a cleft when I say that our mission is to help each individual achieve personal success in their life without special regard to their original malformation. This will only be possible when cleft jaw surgery is readily available to all of those in need.[9]

Letter from a Past Patient (see Fig. 8.9)

Dearest Dr. Posnick,

Every time I try to write this letter, I can't because I truly don't know how to say it! Nothing I say can encompass my gratitude for what you've done for me since I was a baby with a cleft lip and palate. You went above and beyond with your care and always made me feel safe and comfortable which was so important to me. I painted you orchids because that is the flower you always had in your office at the time of my visits. Now whenever I see orchids I am reminded of you and your staff and the kindness shown to me during that bit of my life. The surgeries you performed, especially the jaw surgery, have changed my life dramatically and positively. I am eternally thankful.

Xoxo
Eleanor

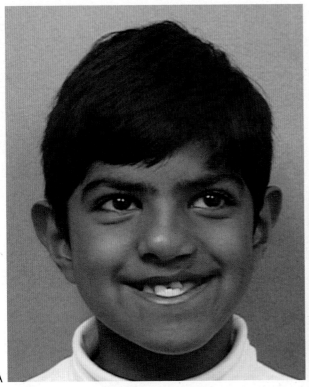

A   7 yrs of age after cleft lip & palate repair

missing lateral incisor - cleft defect - oronasal fistula

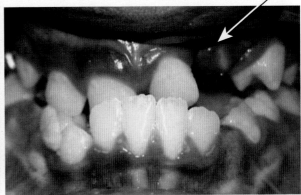

prior to bone grafting cleft & fistula closure

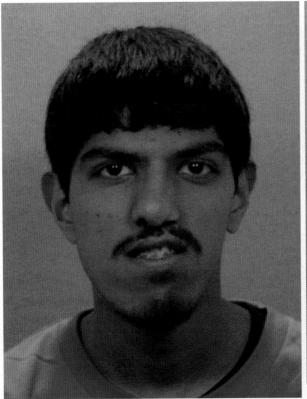

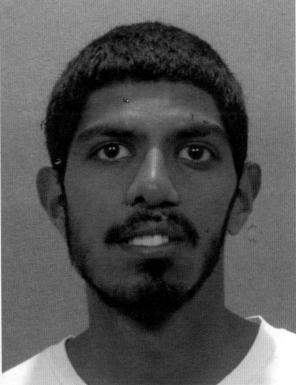

B   teenager before & after cleft jaw & nasal reconstruction

• **Figure 9.1** A child who was born with a complete unilateral cleft lip and palate (UCLP). He underwent primary lip and palate repair at another institution. He was referred to this surgeon and underwent successful mixed dentition bone grafting and fistula closure. As a teenager, he demonstrated cleft maxillary hypoplasia with secondary deformities of the mandible and the nose. He then underwent a coordinated orthodontic and bimaxillary orthognathic surgical approach. The surgery included Le Fort I osteotomy; sagittal (split) ramus osteotomies of the mandible; osseous genioplasty; septoplasty; and inferior turbinate reduction. Six months after jaw surgery, definitive nasal reconstruction including use of a rib cartilage graft was accomplished. **A,** He is shown at 7 years of age just before mixed-dentition bone grafting of the cleft defect. **B,** Frontal views in repose before and after jaw and nasal reconstruction.

Continued

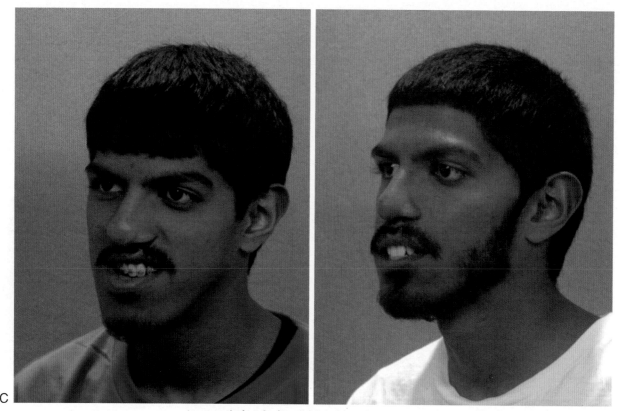

teenager before & after cleft jaw & nasal reconstruction

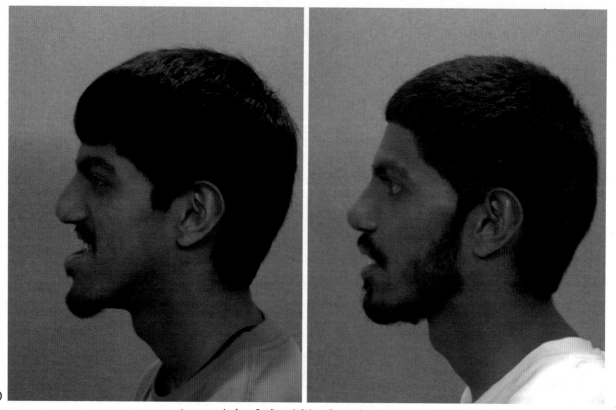

teenager before & after cleft jaw & nasal reconstruction

Figure 9.1, cont'd C, Oblique facial views before and after cleft jaw and nasal reconstruction. **D,** Profile views before and after cleft jaw and nasal reconstruction.

Continued

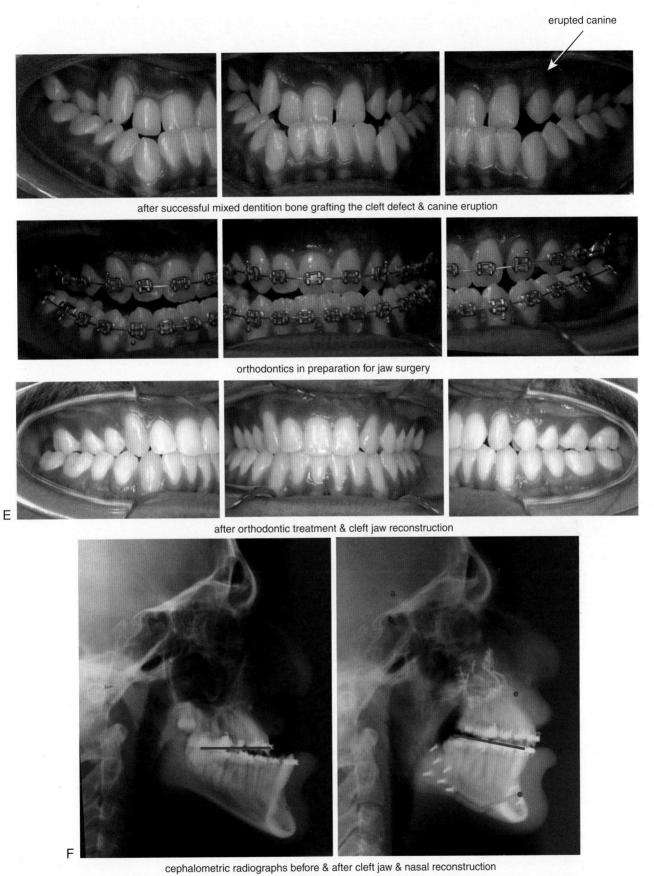

erupted canine

after successful mixed dentition bone grafting the cleft defect & canine eruption

orthodontics in preparation for jaw surgery

E

after orthodontic treatment & cleft jaw reconstruction

F

cephalometric radiographs before & after cleft jaw & nasal reconstruction

Figure 9.1, cont'd E, Occlusal views are shown before and then after the completion of cleft reconstruction. **F,** Cephalometric radiographs before and after cleft reconstruction. (A–F) From Posnick JC. Cleft orthognathic surgery: The unilateral cleft lip and palate deformity. *Orthognathic Surgery: Principles and Practice*, 2nd ed. (JC Posnick, ed., B Kinard, assoc. ed.). St. Louis: Elsevier. Ch. 32, Fig. 32-9, pp. 1313–1316; 2022.

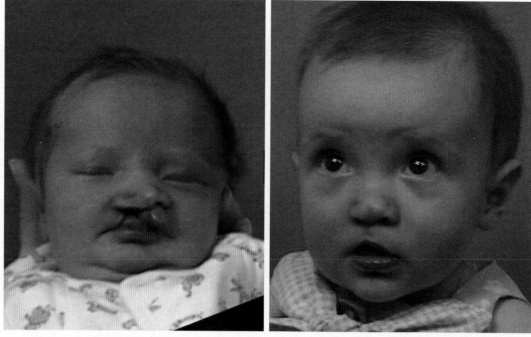

newborn with UCLP   1 week after primary cleft lip repair

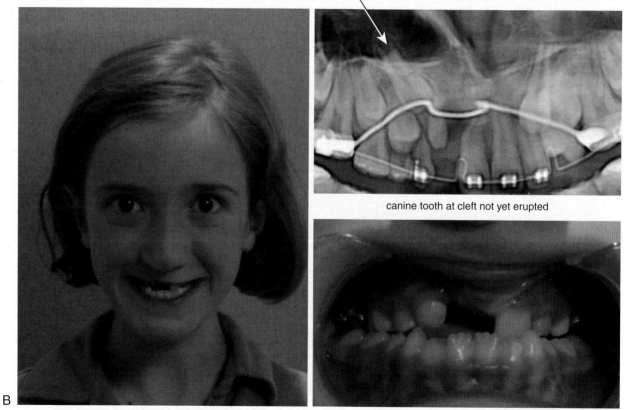

7 years of age after cleft lip & palate repair

canine tooth at cleft not yet erupted

prior to bone grafting cleft & fistula closure

• **Figure 9.2** A child who was born with a complete UCLP. She was referred to this surgeon at birth and underwent primary lip and palate repair during infancy. She underwent successful mixed dentition bone grafting and fistula closure at 7 years of age. As a teenager, she demonstrated cleft maxillary hypoplasia with secondary deformities of the mandible and the nose. She then underwent a coordinated orthodontic and bimaxillary orthognathic surgical approach. The surgery included Le Fort I osteotomy in two segments; sagittal (split) ramus osteotomies of the mandible; osseous genioplasty; septoplasty; and inferior turbinate reduction. Six months after jaw surgery, definitive nasal reconstruction including use of a rib cartilage graft was accomplished. **A,** The patient is shown prior to and early after primary cleft lip repair. **B,** She is shown at 7 years of age, just before mixed-dentition bone grafting. The arrow points to the developing canine tooth at the cleft, not yet erupted.

Continued

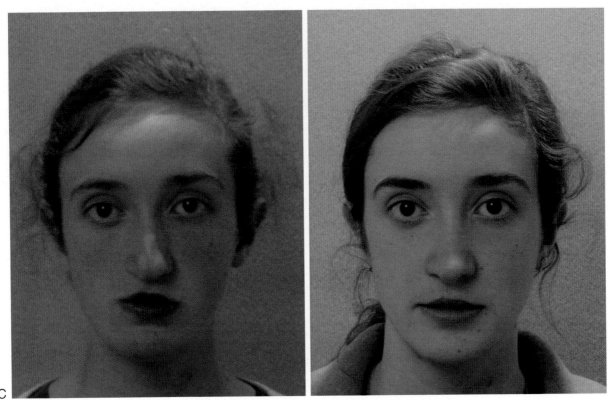

teenager before & after cleft jaw & nasal reconstruction

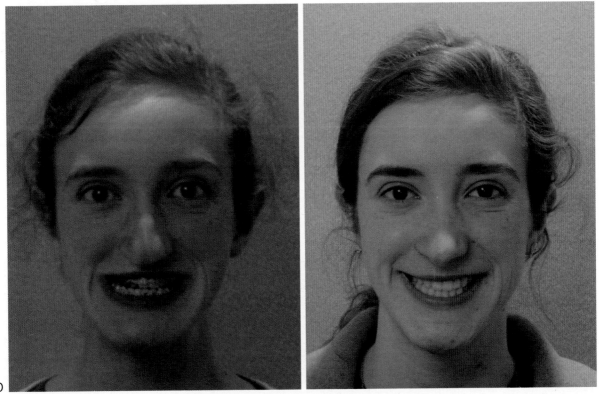

teenager before & after cleft jaw & nasal reconstruction

Figure 9.2, cont'd C, Frontal views in repose before and after jaw and nasal reconstruction. **D,** Frontal views with smile before and after cleft jaw and nasal reconstruction.

Continued

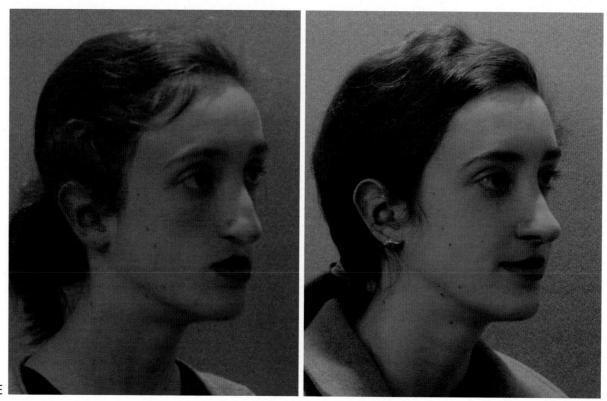

teenager before & after cleft jaw & nasal reconstruction

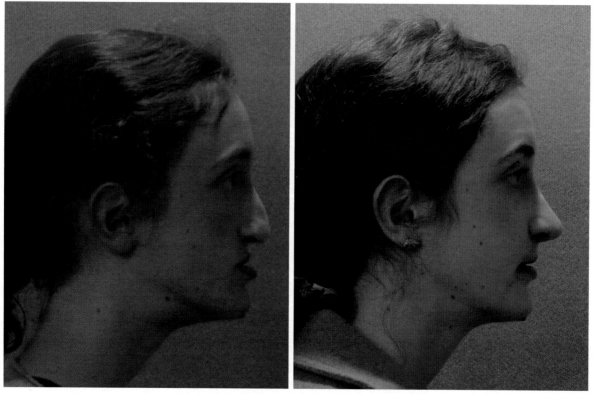

teenager before & after cleft jaw & nasal reconstruction

Figure 9.2, cont'd **E,** Oblique facial views before and after cleft jaw and nasal reconstruction. **F,** Profile views before and after cleft jaw and nasal reconstruction.

Continued

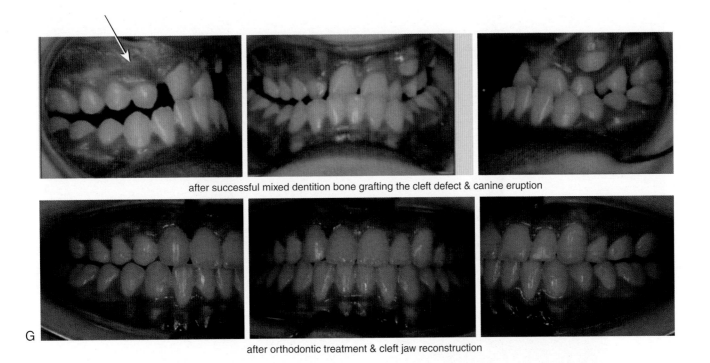

after successful mixed dentition bone grafting the cleft defect & canine eruption

G

after orthodontic treatment & cleft jaw reconstruction

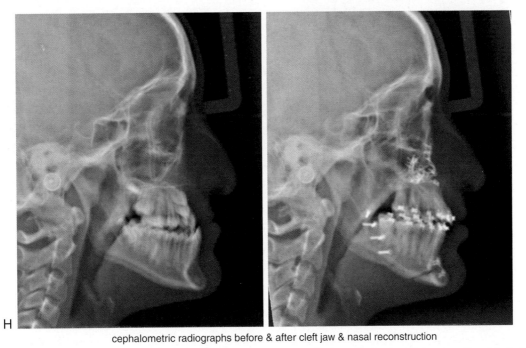

H

cephalometric radiographs before & after cleft jaw & nasal reconstruction

Figure 9.2, cont'd G, Occlusal views before and then after the completion of cleft reconstruction. H, Cephalometric radiographs before and after cleft reconstruction. (A–H) From Posnick JC. Cleft orthognathic surgery: The unilateral cleft lip and palate deformity. *Orthognathic Surgery: Principles and Practice*, 2nd ed. (JC Posnick, ed., B Kinard, assoc. ed.). St. Louis: Elsevier. Ch. 32, Fig. 32-10, pp. 1582–1586; 2022.

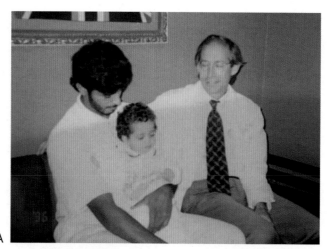

child with cleft lip & palate arrived from UAE for cleft care

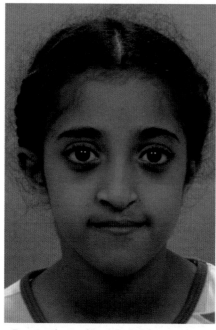

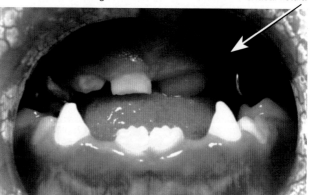

missing lateral incisor - cleft defect - oronasal fistula

B 7 years of age after cleft lip & palate repair

prior to bone grafting cleft & fistula closure

• **Figure 9.3** A child who was born with left-sided UCLP. She was referred to this surgeon, arriving from the UAE, and underwent primary lip and palate repair during infancy. She underwent successful mixed-dentition grafting and fistula closure at 7 years of age. As a teenager, she underwent a coordinated orthodontic and bimaxillary orthognathic approach. The surgery included Le Fort I osteotomy in two segments; sagittal (split) ramus osteotomies of the mandible; osseous genioplasty; septoplasty; and inferior turbinate reduction. Six months after jaw surgery, nasal reconstruction including use of a rib cartilage graft was accomplished. **A,** Surgeon with father and child on arrival to hospital for cleft care. **B,** She is shown at 7 years of age, just before mixed-dentition bone grafting. The arrow points to the developing canine tooth at the cleft, not yet erupted.

Continued

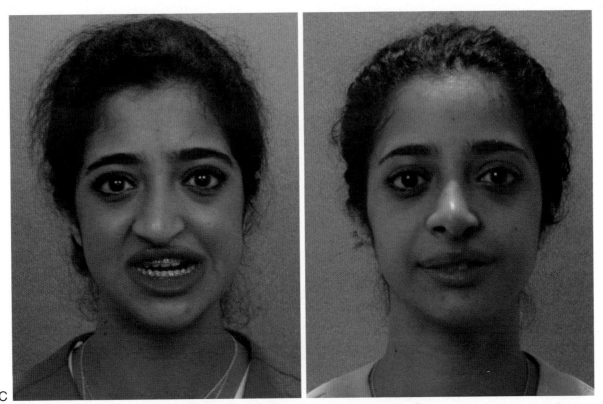

teenager before & after cleft jaw & nasal reconstruction

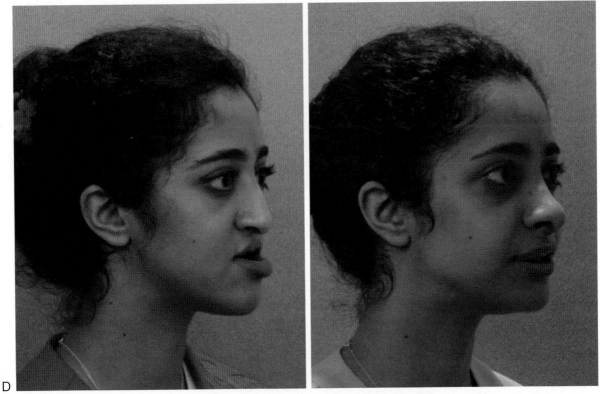

teenager before & after cleft jaw & nasal reconstruction

Figure 9.3, cont'd C, Frontal views with smile before and after cleft reconstruction. D, Oblique facial views before and after cleft reconstruction.

Continued

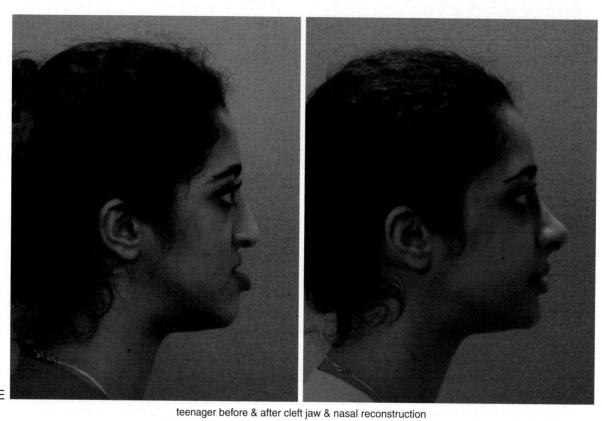

teenager before & after cleft jaw & nasal reconstruction

Figure 9.3, cont'd **E,** Profile views before and after cleft reconstruction.

Continued

erupted canine

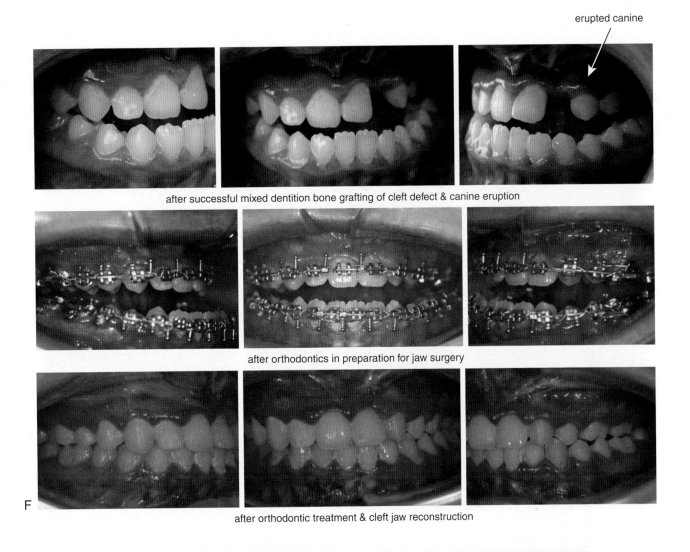

after successful mixed dentition bone grafting of cleft defect & canine eruption

after orthodontics in preparation for jaw surgery

F

after orthodontic treatment & cleft jaw reconstruction

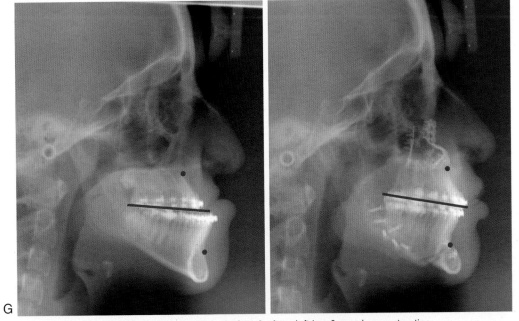

G

cephalometric radiographs before & after cleft jaw & nasal reconstruction

Figure 9.3, cont'd F, Occlusal views are shown before orthodontics, with orthodontics in preparation for orthognathic surgery, and after the completion of reconstruction. **G,** Cephalometric radiographs before and after reconstruction.

Continued

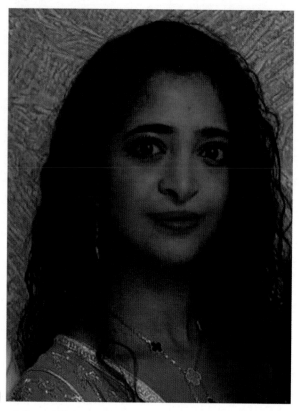

Hello Professor Posnick,

I am so happy that I had the chance to be your patient since I was a little baby. I am thankful for everything you did to me throughout the years. From the bottom of my heart I wish you all the happiness in this life as you are one of the reasons I am who I am.

Hessa

H

Figure 9.3, cont'd H, She is shown at 25 years of age, now working as an accountant back home in the UAE. (A–H) From Posnick JC. Cleft orthognathic surgery: The unilateral cleft lip and palate deformity. *Orthognathic Surgery: Principles and Practice*, 2nd ed. (JC Posnick, ed., B Kinard, assoc. ed.). St. Louis: Elsevier. Ch. 32, Fig. 32-12, pp. 1593–1597; 2022.

References

1. Parameters for evaluation and treatment of patients with cleft lip/palate or other craniofacial differences. *Cleft Palate Craniofac J.* 2017;55(1):137–156.
2. Good PM, Mulliken JB, Padwa BL. Le Fort I osteotomy after repaired CL/P or CP. *Cleft Palate Craniofac J.* 2007;44:396.
3. Obwegeser HL. *Surgical correction of deformities of the jaws in adult cleft cases.* Houston, Texas: Paper read at the First International Conference on Cleft Lip and Palate; 1969:14–17.
4. Posnick JC, Tompson B. Cleft-orthognathic surgery: complications and long-term results. *Plast Reconstr Surg.* 1995;96(2):255–266.
5. Posnick JC, Kinard BE. Challenges in the successful reconstruction of cleft lip and palate: managing the nasomaxillary deformity in adolescence. *Plast Reconstr Surg.* 2020;145:591e.
6. Posnick JC, Kinard BE. Reconstruction of residual cleft nasal deformities using a rib cartilage caudal strut graft: diagnosis and surgical approach. *Otorhinolaryngol Head Neck Surg.* 2019;4:1–5.
7. Posnick JC, Susarla SM, Kinard BE. Reconstruction of residual cleft nasal deformities in adolescents: effects on social perceptions. *J Craniomaxillofac Surg.* 2019;47:1414–1419.
8. Posnick JC, Susarla SM, Kinard BE. The effect of cleft orthognathic and nasal reconstruction on perceived social traits. *Plast Reconstr Surg Glob Open.* 2019;7:e2422.
9. Posnick JC, Kinard BE. Why do only 15% of adolescents in the US with a cleft jaw deformity undergo reconstruction? *Cleft Palate Craniofac J.* 2021;58(5):644–646.

10

Reconstruction of Hemifacial Microsomia

JEFFREY C. POSNICK, DMD, MD

Hemifacial microsomia (HFM) is a term used to describe a condition that occurs during embryological development and results in a deficiency (hypoplasia) of tissues within the face. This malformation may affect the spectrum of structures located within the first and second branchial arches of the face (e.g., skeleton, skin, muscles, nerves, glands, teeth). The cranial vault (i.e., the bones that surround and protect the brain), orbit (i.e., the bones that surround and protect the eye), cheekbone, and even the eye may also have structural deficiencies (see Figs. 10.1 and 10.2). It typically affects just one side of the face and may even result in clefting through the corner of the mouth (see Fig. 10.3). Hemifacial microsomia will always have major effects on the jaws and the external ear (see Figs. 10.4 and 10.5). The hemifacial microsomia malformation is expected to have potential functional consequences on the child's vision, hearing, breathing, speech articulation, chewing ability, and, over time, on self-esteem.

Despite over half a century of attempts to standardize the effective reconstruction of this relatively common malformation (1/5000 newborns), much confusion and disagreement in the medical and dental literature remains.[1–4] Reconstruction of deformities of the external ear and of the jaws remain inconsistently treated with variable and often suboptimal functional and aesthetic results.[4,5]

Once the affected child's jaw growth approaches maturity (13–15 years of age), orthodontics can properly reposition the teeth and then the jaws can be reconstructed through planned osteotomies and the use of bone grafts.[1,3] The goal of skeletal reconstruction is to 3-dimensionally reconfigure the hypoplastic structures for optimal form and function (see Figs. 10.2 and 10.4).

Achieving an open airway, improved speech articulation, chewing ability and occlusion, as well as a pleasing facial appearance that no longer draws negative attention to the individual, is the objective of treatment. Completion of reconstruction and dental rehabilitation for the teenager, prior to their high school graduation, should be accomplished. Clearly, more work needs to be done to achieve a successful reconstruction for all affected children.

Letter from a Past Patient

Dear Dr. Posnick,

Thank you so much for all that you have done for me over the past few years. When you first met me, I was much younger and with my parents. Until the facial and jaw surgeries, I felt ashamed of my face and smile, but now I feel much more confident in my relationships and daily life. Your commitment to my well-being has truly changed my life and I cannot stress how much I appreciate it.

Love,
Christina Jackson

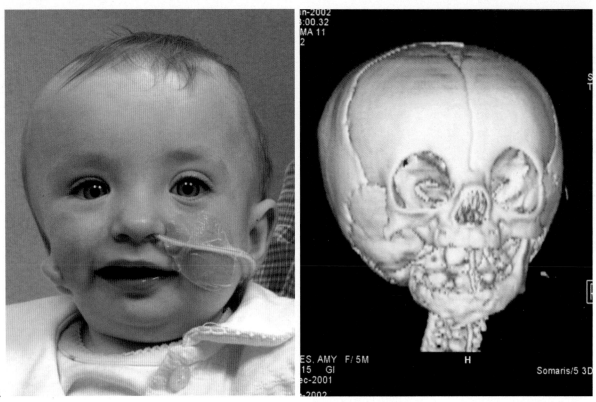

newborn with right sided hemifacial microsomia

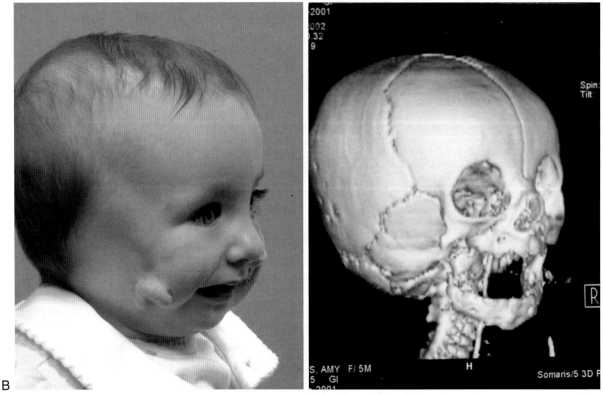

newborn with right sided hemifacial microsomia

• **Figure 10.1** A newborn child with a right sided HFM. **A–C,** Facial and CT scan views. The extent of the soft tissue in skeletal deficiencies of the structures within the first and second branchial arches is shown. On the right side of the face, the cranial vault (skull) and the orbit (the bone surrounding the eye) are hypoplastic (small). The cheekbone is absent. The maxilla is small and the mandible is partially absent and small. All of the soft tissues on the right side of the face are also hypoplastic and the right ear and ear canal are absent. (A–C) From Posnick JC. Hemifacial microsomia: Evaluation and treatment. *Orthognathic Surgery: Principles and Practice*, 2nd ed. (JC Posnick, ed., B Kinard, assoc. ed.). St. Louis: Elsevier. Chapter 28, Fig. 28-6, pp. 1338–1339; 2022.

Continued

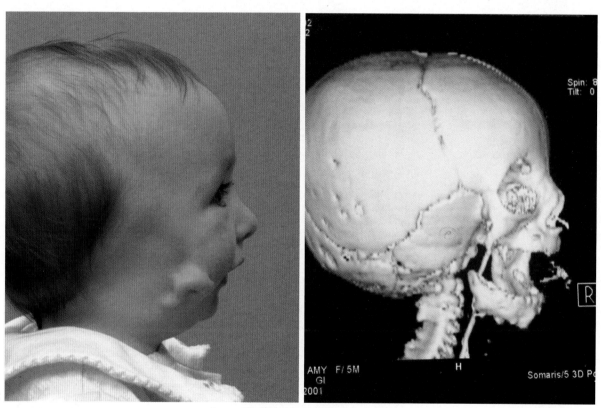

C

newborn with right sided hemifacial microsomia

Figure 10.1, cont'd

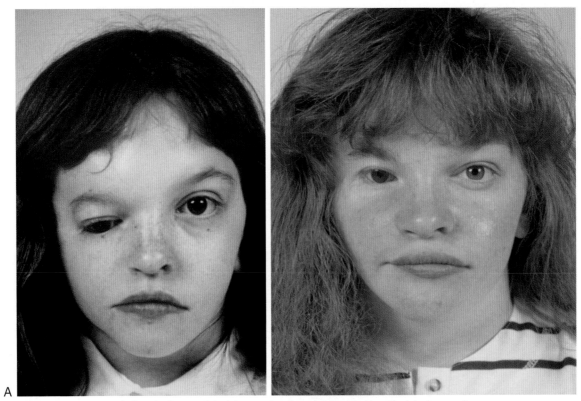

before & after craniofacial reconstruction of right sided hemifacial microsomia

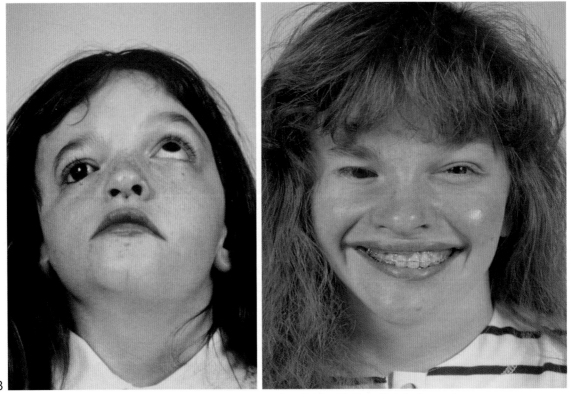

before & after craniofacial reconstruction of right sided hemifacial microsomia

• **Figure 10.2** A girl who was born with a right sided HFM that included extensive involvement of the upper facial skeleton, micro-ophthalmia (missing eye), the lower facial skeleton (missing parts of the mandible), and microtia (absent external ear). She had undergone several intracranial cranio-orbital procedures at another institution with limited success. She was referred to this surgeon at 10 years of age and underwent two definitive reconstructive procedures. The first included a transcranial approach, including osteotomies and bone grafting to reconstruct the cranial vault, the right orbit, and the right cheekbone. The second procedure was to correct the jaw deformities, including a Le Fort I osteotomy, sagittal (split) ramus osteotomies of the mandible, and an osseous genioplasty in combination with orthodontics. She is shown at 10 years of age prior to and then at 15 years of age after the two operations. **A,** Frontal views in repose before and after reconstruction. **B,** Worm's-eye view before surgery and frontal view with smile after reconstruction.

Continued

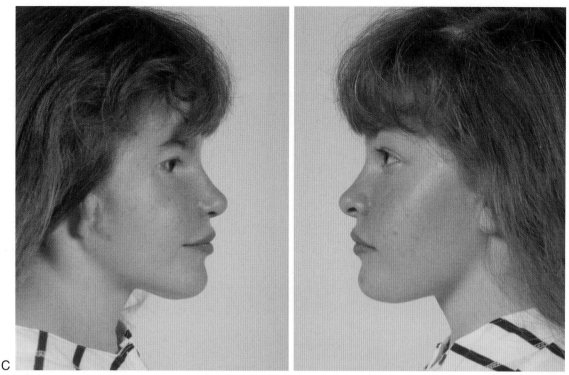

C profile views of facial symmetry after right sided craniofacial reconstruction

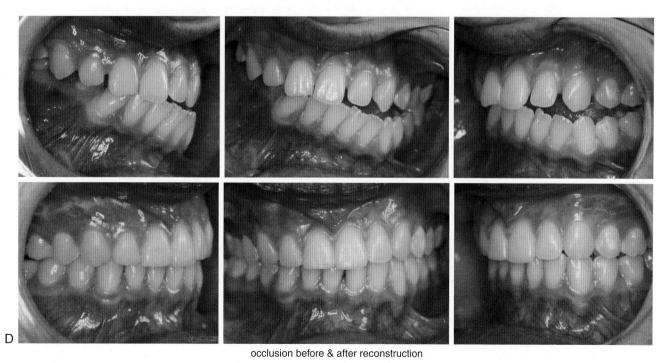

D occlusion before & after reconstruction

Figure 10.2, cont'd C, Right and left profile views after reconstruction of the right side of the face indicating achieved facial symmetry. D, Occlusal views before and after reconstruction.

Continued

congenital hypoplasia of cranial vault, orbit, & cheekbone

reconstruction complete

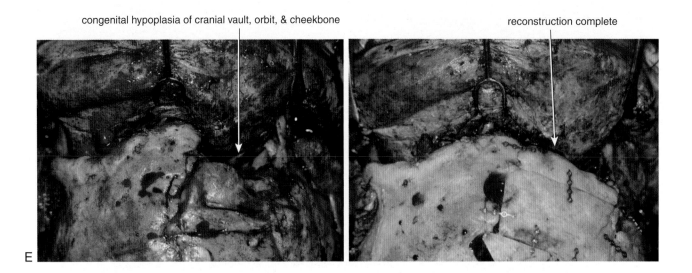

E

before & after cranial vault, orbital & cheekbone reconstruction

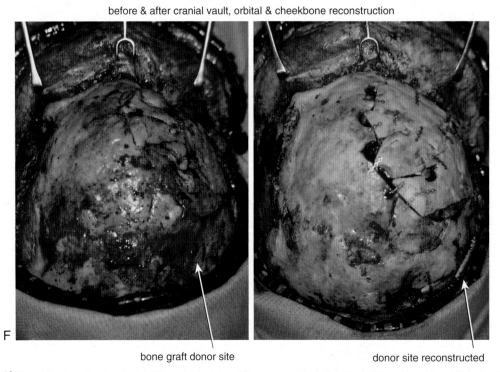

F

bone graft donor site

donor site reconstructed

Figure 10.2, cont'd E and F, Intraoperative views of the cranial vault and the upper orbits before and after redo cranio-orbital zygomatic reconstruction. (A–F) From Posnick JC. Hemifacial microsomia: Evaluation and staging of reconstruction. *J Oral Maxillofac Surg.* 1998;56:648.

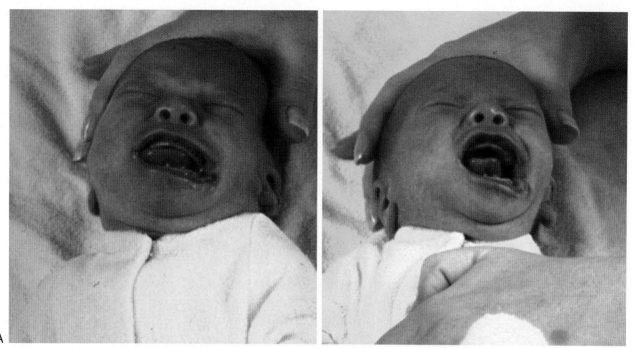

newborn with left sided hemifacial microsomia & cleft of left oral commissure

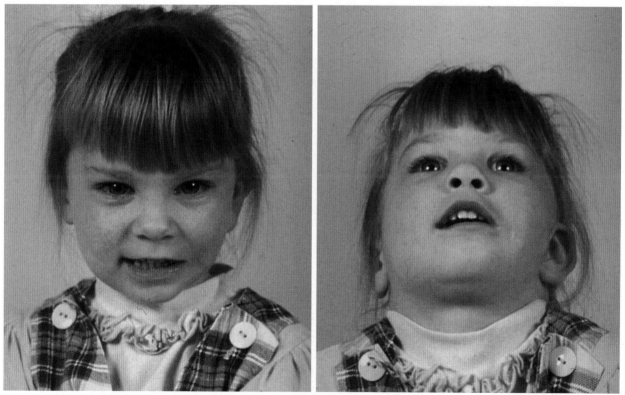

1 yr after repair of left oral commissure

• **Figure 10.3** A newborn with a mild form of HFM, also including macrostomia (clefting) of the left oral commissure. She is shown before and 1 year after macrostomia repair. **A,** Facial views before macrostomia repair. **B,** Facial views after oral commissure reconstruction. (A–B) From Posnick JC. Hemifacial microsomia: Evaluation and treatment. *Orthognathic Surgery: Principles and Practice*, 2nd ed. (JC Posnick, ed., B Kinard, assoc. ed.). St. Louis: Elsevier. Ch. 28, Fig. 28-1, p. 1330; 2022.

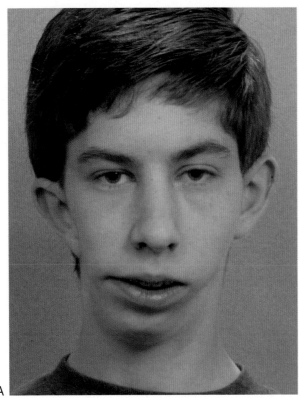

A

teenager with right sided hemifacial microsomia

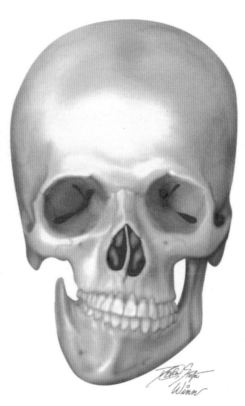

illustration of hemifacial microsomia deformity

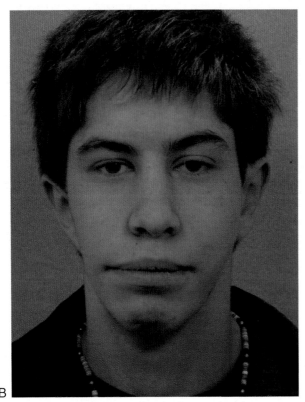

B

after jaw reconstruction & ear setback

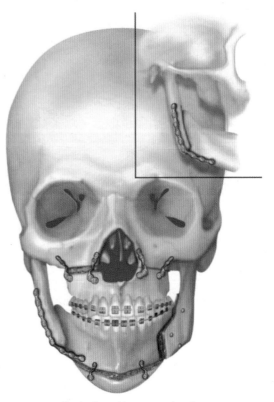

illustration of jaw reconstruction

• **Figure 10.4** A boy who was born with a right sided HFM. There was a type IIB mandibular malformation (i.e., missing the condyle of the lower jaw). The patient was followed longitudinally without treatment intervention until he approached skeletal maturity. After the patient was in the adult dentition non-extraction orthodontic treatment and single-stage reconstruction that included Le Fort I osteotomy in two segments; left-sided sagittal (split) ramus osteotomy; right mandibular construction with a rib graft; osseous genioplasty; and bilateral ear setback. **A,** Frontal facial view prior to surgery and illustration of the presenting skeletal deformities. **B,** Frontal facial view after surgery and illustration of the reconstruction that was carried out.

Continued

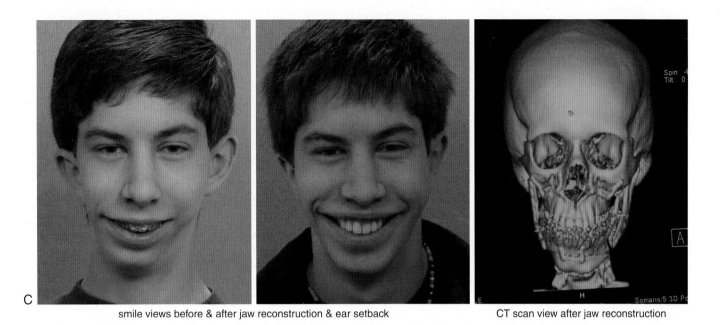

smile views before & after jaw reconstruction & ear setback   CT scan view after jaw reconstruction

occlusion before & after jaw reconstruction with rib graft

Figure 10.4, cont'd C, Frontal views with smile before and after reconstruction. 3-D CT scan view after reconstruction. **D,** Occlusal views with orthodontics in progress and after reconstruction.

Continued

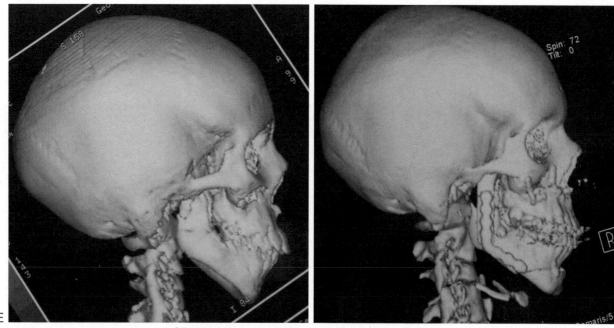

CT scan views before & after jaw reconstruction with rib graft

Figure 10.4, cont'd **E,** Profile CT scan views before and after reconstruction that indicate rib graft reconstruction. (A–E) From Posnick JC. Hemifacial microsomia: Evaluation and treatment. *Orthognathic Surgery: Principles and Practice*, 2nd ed. (JC Posnick, ed., B Kinard, assoc. ed.). St. Louis: Elsevier. Ch. 28, Fig. 28-16, pp. 1383–1387; 2022.

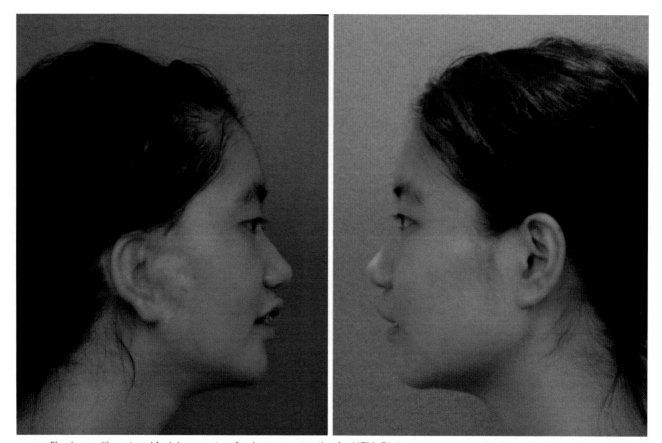

profile views with restored facial symmetry after jaw reconstruction for HFM. Right ear reconstructed using polyethylene framework

• **Figure 10.5** An 18-year-old Asian female with a right sided HFM. She underwent microtia (external ear) reconstruction with a porous polyethylene framework (at another institution) at 7 years of age. She is shown at 18 years of age, 5 weeks after undergoing single stage jaw reconstruction by this surgeon. The procedures included Le Fort I osteotomy in two segments; left-sided sagittal (split) ramus osteotomy; right mandibular construction with a rib graft; and osseous genioplasty. Note: The purpose of showing this HFM patient is primarily to demonstrate the favorable microtia (external ear) reconstruction. From Posnick JC. Hemifacial microsomia: Evaluation and treatment. *Orthognathic Surgery: Principles and Practice*, 2nd ed. (JC Posnick, ed., B Kinnard, assoc. ed.). St. Louis: Elsevier. Ch. 28, Fig. 28-17, p. 1390; 2022.

References

1. Kaban LB, Padwa BL, Mulliken JB. Surgical correction of mandibular hypoplasia in hemifacial microsomia: the case for treatment in early childhood. *J Oral Maxillofac Surg.* 1998;56(5):628–638.

2. Brent B. Advances in ear reconstruction with autogenous rib cartilage grafts: personal experience with 1200 cases. *Plast Reconstr Surg.* 1999;104:319.

3. Posnick JC. Hemifacial microsomia: evaluation and staging of reconstruction. *J Oral Maxillofac Surg.* 1998;56:648.

4. Posnick JC. Hemifacial microsomia: evaluation and treatment. In: Posnick JC, ed., Kinard B, assoc. ed. *Orthognathic Surgery: Principles and Practice.* 2nd ed. St. Louis: Elsevier; 2022. ch. 28.

5. Hamlet C, Harcourt D. Exploring the experiences of adults with microtia: a qualitative study. *Cleft Palate Craniofac J.* 2020;57(10):1230–1237.

11

Reconstruction of Posttraumatic Jaw Deformities

JEFFREY C. POSNICK, DMD, MD

Despite the best efforts of primary care physicians and hospital-based trauma teams, a subgroup of children who sustain facial injuries later present with secondary deformities that require reconstruction. In the pediatric patient, even with optimal primary treatment, if the injured and repaired maxillofacial structures do not continue to grow normally (and often they do not) secondary deformities result. Teeth may also have been lost or displaced as part of the original injury and soft tissue lacerations may have healed with permanent scars.

The causes of a facial injury in childhood run the gamut including falls, sports accidents, pedestrian injuries, motor vehicle accidents, animal bites, and gunshot wounds. Injured facial structures in children, as opposed to adults, have the added requirement of need for ongoing growth. The injured bones and the not yet fully formed teeth may be traumatically inhibited from reaching their full potential. The occurrence of these secondary jaw growth disturbances is not a new nor a unique problem. In 1909, Dr. Vilray Blair reported in the *Journal of the American Medical Association* his experience with a 21-year-old woman who arrived for evaluation with a secondary (posttraumatic) jaw deformity including fusion of the jaw joints (temporomandibular joint [TMJ] ankylosis). This was after she had sustained lower jaw trauma in childhood. Blair stated: "A young woman was referred to me and gave the following history. When five years of age she was crushed under a falling bale of hay. [She] remained unconscious for 48 hours, but [then] made a good recovery. Between the ages of 11–12 years, it was noticed that she could not open her mouth freely. On examination it was found that the range of movement of the lower jaw was limited. From that time on, the chin became more receded. Owing to the receded jaw, the lower teeth were [very much] behind the upper [teeth]. I thought that the lack of [jaw] development was related to the earlier injury." In 1907, under general anesthesia, Blair "made neck incisions, sawed through the lower jaw on each side to release the [TMJ] ankylosis and then advanced the mandible". He stated: "Unfortunately, there was limited improvement in the [woman's] profile and the [TMJ] ankylosis reoccurred."[1] Fortunately, we have made great strides in posttraumatic jaw reconstruction since Blair's time.

Thoughtfully timed posttraumatic jaw reconstruction, coordinated with orthodontic and dental treatment, must consider the individual's functional needs (i.e., breathing, chewing, speech), psychosocial concerns (i.e., self-esteem, body image), and skeletal maturity (see Figs. 11.1 and 11.2).[2-5] The treatment should be individualized with the objective to provide successful reconstruction and dental rehabilitation prior to the teenager graduating from high school. Unfortunately, the reconstructive potential for these posttraumatic deformities in children may be misunderstood and therefore neglected. In the future, specialized facial surgeons and dental specialists in each major metropolitan community will be trained and available to correct these complex deformities.

Letter from a Past Patient

Dear Dr. Posnick,

I'm writing to let you know how thrilled I am with the results of my jaw surgery. Before, because of the car accident, when looking in the mirror no matter what I did I no longer felt attractive. Now I am again proud of my facial profile and my teeth alignment. For the first time in a long time I feel beautiful in all ways and can also chew without difficulty. I never thought that would again be possible. I'm grateful for the confidence the surgery has given me. Thanks again for everything you have done.

Sincerely,
Susan Gunderson

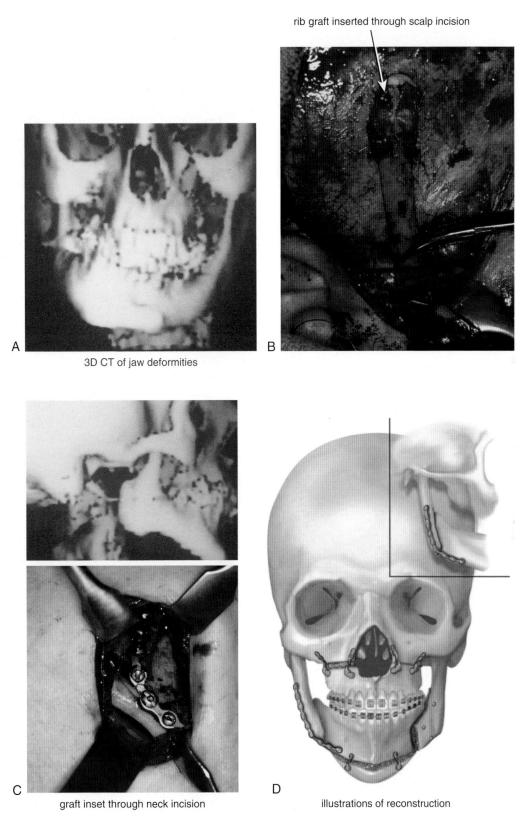

rib graft inserted through scalp incision

A

3D CT of jaw deformities

B

C

graft inset through neck incision

D

illustrations of reconstruction

• **Figure 11.1** A 16-year-old boy who had sustained a displaced right condylar neck fracture of the mandible during early childhood. He presented to this surgeon after resorption of the condylar fracture fragment and with a resulting facial asymmetry. He agreed to jaw reconstruction to improve the facial asymmetry, correct the unstable bite, and the limited mouth opening. The reconstruction included Le Fort I osteotomy, left sagittal (split) ramus osteotomy, construction of the right condyle–ramus unit with a rib graft, and osseous genioplasty. **A,** The computed tomography (CT) scans confirm an absent right condyle and the extent of facial asymmetry that affects the maxilla and mandible. **B,** The intraoperative view demonstrates insertion of the rib graft through a scalp incision as a component of the reconstruction. **C,** Graft stabilization is with a titanium mini-plate and screws placed through a neck incision. **D,** Illustration of the overall reconstruction.

Continued

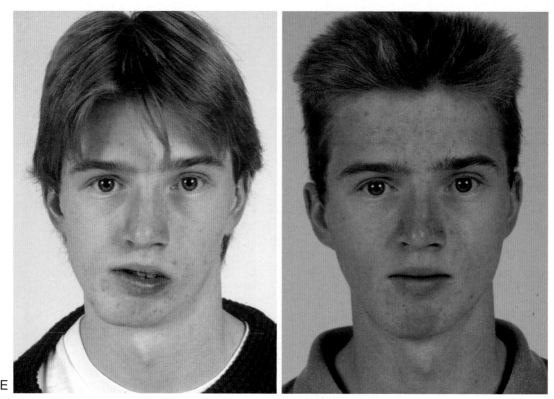

teenager before & after posttraumatic jaw reconstruction

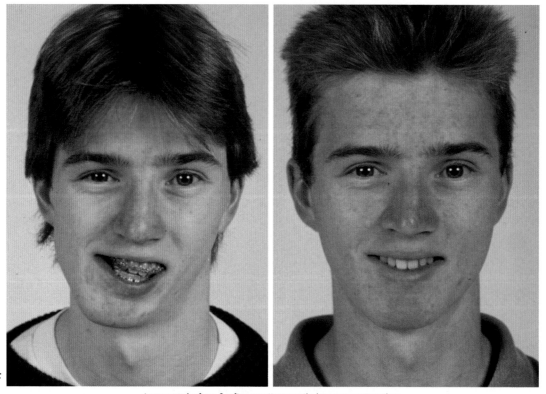

teenager before & after posttraumatic jaw reconstruction

Figure 11.1, cont'd **E,** Frontal views in repose before and after reconstruction. **F,** Frontal views with smile before and after reconstruction.

Continued

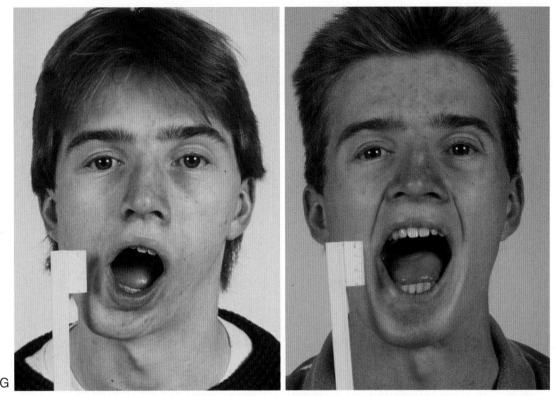

teenager before & after posttraumatic jaw reconstruction

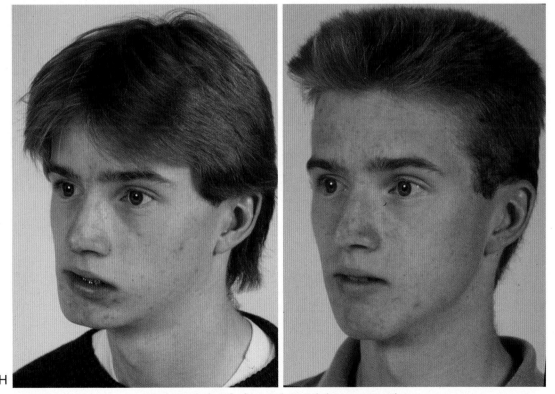

teenager before & after posttraumatic jaw reconstruction

Figure 11.1, cont'd G, Improved mouth opening after reconstruction. **H,** Oblique facial views before and after reconstruction.

Continued

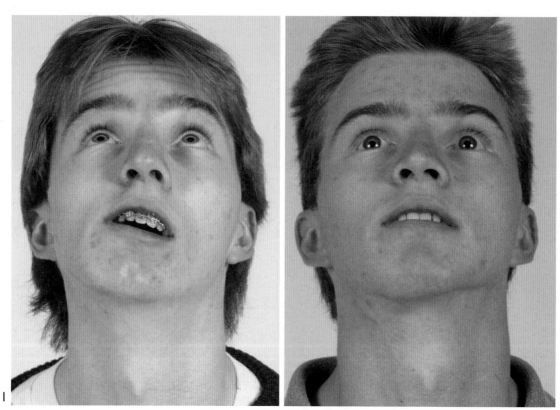

teenager before & after posttraumatic jaw reconstruction

Figure 11.1, cont'd I, Worm's-eye views before and after reconstruction. (A–I) From Posnick JC. Management of facial fractures in children and adolescents. *Ann Plast Surg.* 1994;33(4):442–457.

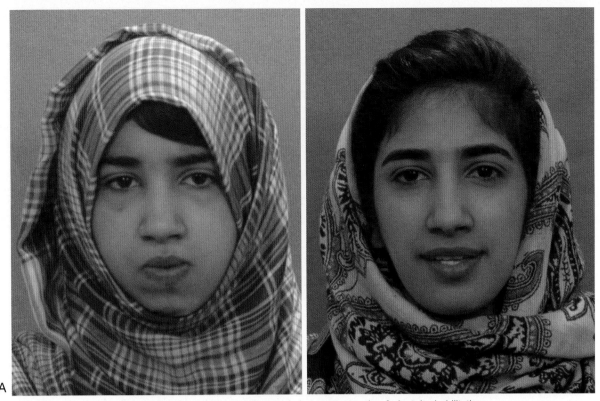

teenager before & after posttraumatic jaw reconstruction & dental rehabilitation

A

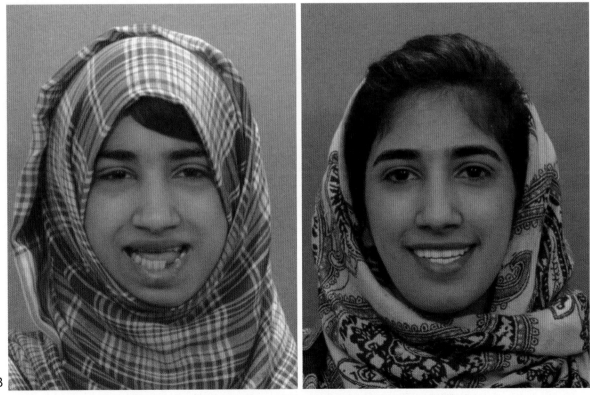

teenager before & after posttraumatic jaw reconstruction & dental rehabilitation

B

• **Figure 11.2** At 16 years of age, this teenager fell from a height of 6 meters and sustained maxillofacial and lower extremity trauma. Her maxillofacial injuries included displaced left and right condyle fractures, a comminuted left parasymphyseal fracture of the mandible with the loss of teeth, and anterior maxillary fracture with loss of teeth. She was treated at another institution with tracheostomy, open treatment of the comminuted parasymphyseal fracture, debridement of the anterior maxilla and associated teeth, and closed treatment of the bilateral condyle fractures. She was referred to this surgeon when she was 20 years old for secondary reconstruction. She was found to have bilateral TMJ ankylosis, malunion of the mandible, an anterior maxillary dentoalveolar defect with loss of multiple teeth in both jaws. Staged maxillofacial reconstruction and dental rehabilitation included left and right TMJ ankylosis release (gap arthroplasty) with documented sustained improved mandibular opening. Six months later, maxillo-mandibular reconstruction included: sagittal (split) ramus osteotomies of the mandible; left parasymphyseal osteotomy; oblique osteotomy of the chin; anterior maxillary dentoalveolar defect reconstruction with a hip graft; and revision of the tracheostomy scar. Six months after successful jaw reconstruction, four dental implants were placed. This was followed 6 months later with restorative dentistry, including crown and bridge reconstruction in both jaws. **A,** Frontal views in repose before and after reconstruction and dental rehabilitation. **B,** Frontal views with smile before and after reconstruction and dental rehabilitation.

Continued

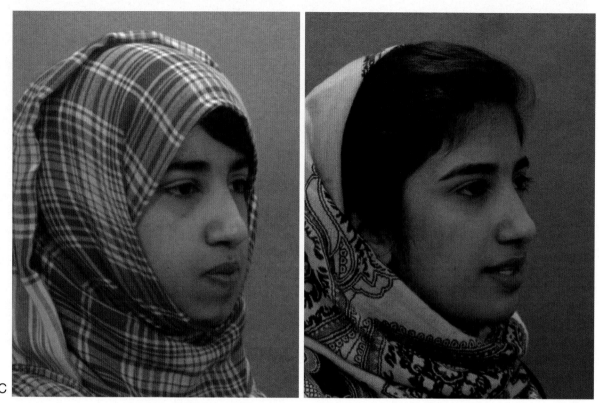

teenager before & after posttraumatic jaw reconstruction & dental rehabilitation

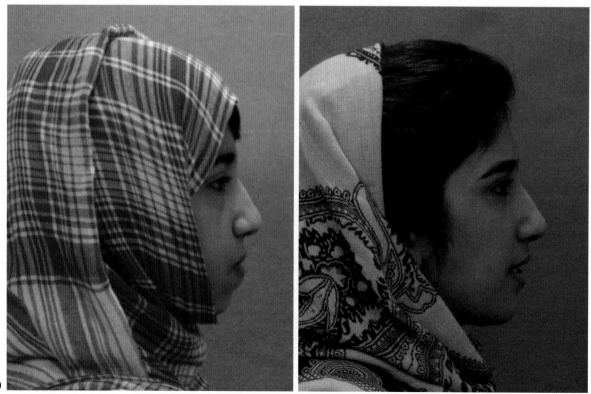

before & after posttraumatic jaw reconstruction & dental reconstruction

Figure 11.2, cont'd **C,** Oblique facial views before and after reconstruction and dental rehabilitation. **D,** Profile facial views before and after reconstruction and dental rehabilitation.

Continued

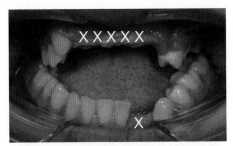

6 missing teeth

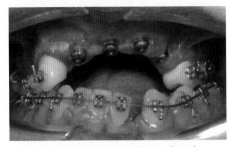

4 maxillary dental implants placed

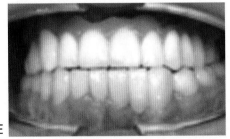

E

dental rehabilitation complete

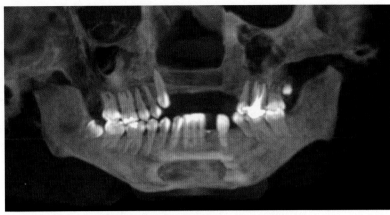

s/p TMJ ankylosis release - gap arthroplasty

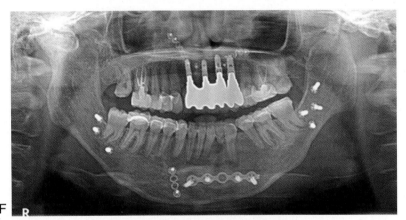

F

after reconstruction/dental rehabilitation

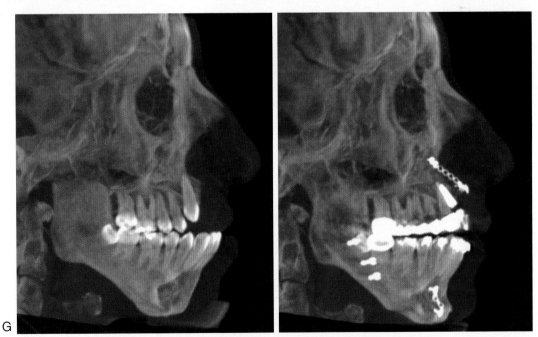

G

cephalometric radiographs before & after posttraumatic jaw reconstruction

Figure 11.2, cont'd **E,** Occlusal views before secondary reconstruction: then after TMJ ankylosis release, bone grafting of the anterior maxilla, and the placement of four dental implants; and finally, after completion of dental rehabilitation. **F,** Panoramic radiographs after ankylosis release (gap arthroplasty) and then after the completion of reconstruction and dental rehabilitation. **G,** Lateral cephalometric radiographs before and after ankylosis release, bone grafting, and mandibular osteotomies. (A–G) From Posnick JC. Management of Secondary Deformities after Maxillofacial Trauma. *Orthognathic Surgery: Principles and Practice*, 2nd ed. (JC Posnick, ed., B Kinard, assoc. ed.). St. Louis: Elsevier. Ch. 35, Fig. 35-9, p. 1828–1831; 2022.

Dear Dr. Posnick,

I want to thank you for giving me a second chance in life. At the age of 11, I was severely injured in a car accident where the left side of my face, including the eye area, was fractured. Even though I was just a child at the time and now I'm in my mid-thirties, I still have not forgotten the miracle procedure you have performed on me. I also remember the follow-up meetings with you. You had a warm smile and reassured me that everything would be fine. I feel fortunate to have had you as my surgeon over 20 years ago and am forever grateful for the gift of a beautiful smile and the confidence that you gave me.

Sincerely,
Julia Chung

References

1. Blair VP. Underdeveloped lower jaw with limited excursion. report of two cases with operation. *J Am Med Assoc*. 1900;53:178.
2. Kaban LB, Perrott DH, Fisher K. A protocol for management of temporomandibular joint ankylosis. *J Oral Maxillofac Surg*. 1990;48:1145.
3. Obwegeser HL. Orthognathic surgery and a tale of how three procedures came to be: a letter to the next generations of surgeons. *Clin Plast Surg*. 2007;34:331–355.
4. Posnick JC. Management of facial fractures in children and adolescents. *Ann Plast Surg*. 1994;33(4):442–457.
5. Posnick JC. Management of secondary jaw deformities after maxillofacial trauma. In: Posnick JC, ed., Kinard B, assoc. ed. *Orthognathic Surgery: Principles and Practice*. 2nd ed. St. Louis: Elsevier; 2022. ch. 35.

12

Reconstruction of Saddle Nose Deformities

JEFFREY C. POSNICK, DMD, MD

The phrase "saddle nose" is a slang term that is still used to describe severe depression of the middle part of the nose when viewed in profile. The term was coined in the late 1800s as it was thought to resemble the concave appearance in the center of a horse's saddle. In those days, the deformity was not an uncommon finding after being kicked in the face by a horse. In 1891, Dr. Roe's reporting of the occurrence of a saddle nose deformity was as follows: "a gentleman was out one day on horseback. His horse, being very spirited, suddenly shied at a piece of paper flying in the street and threw [the man] violently to the ground, directly under the horse's feet. The horse at the same time struck him with a shoe cork of one of its forefeet, directly in the center of the top of his nose, producing a very severe fracture. The nasal bones having been destroyed – the support to the bridge of the nose [was] completely undermined [resulting in a saddle nose]."[1] Subsequently, a succession of surgeons, Weir in the United States (1892), Israel in Germany (1896), and then Joseph, also in Germany (1931), described some success augmenting the depressed nasal bones with bone grafts, sometimes taken from a duck's sternum.[2–4]

These days, saddle nose deformities are more commonly seen in a child after a bicycle fall or after running "nose first" into the edge of a hard, low-set table. Presently, experienced surgeons have become more sophisticated in dissecting the nasal soft tissue envelope, using autogenous grafts, stabilization of the grafts, and then rearranging the cartilage framework of the patient's nose.[5–7] A surgeon's mastery of the artistic aspects of a "saddle nose" reconstruction remain essential in the achievement of functional and aesthetic goals (see Fig. 12.1).

The nasal reconstruction is carried out under general anesthesia, often on an outpatient basis, depending on graft harvesting needs. In the future, reliable manufactured bone and cartilage substitutes and computer-simulated planning should make this reconstruction more accessible for all those in need.

Letter from a Past Patient (see Fig. 12.1)

Dr. Posnick,

You probably don't remember me but I remember you. Now with the internet I was able to find you to say thank you. After an accident when I was child, I couldn't breathe well and my nose was flat. I grew up in Toronto and my parents found you to fix my nose. After the surgery I was fine. I now live in Florida where I go to college and don't think about my nose. Since the surgery it's just like nothing had ever happened. I am sending a picture of me so you can see for yourself. I hope that I get to meet you one day to thank you in person.

Your sincerely,
Neal Kenny

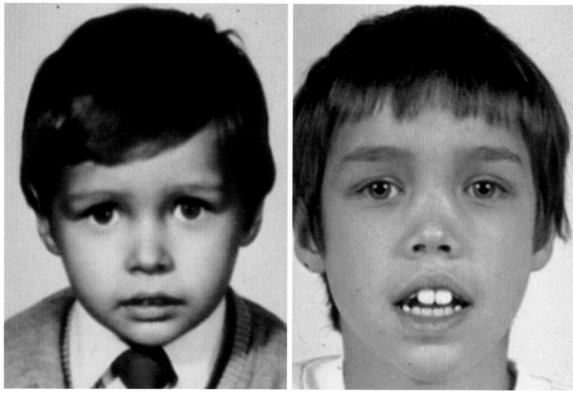

A

3 yrs of age: prior to injury   8 yrs of age: 4 years after "saddle nose" injury

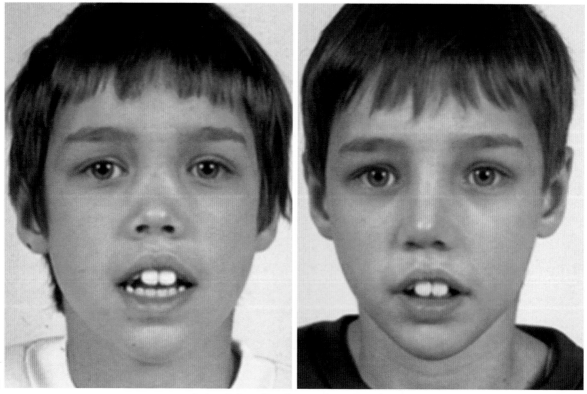

B

before & 6 months after nasal reconstruction

• **Figure 12.1** A 4-year-old boy fell and hit the bridge of his nose on a hard table. Over the next several years, a saddle deformity developed. He was referred to this surgeon when he was 8 years old. The reconstruction included nasal osteotomies; the placement of fixed full-thickness cranial grafts; and repair/securing of the lower lateral cartilages over the top of the graft. **A,** Frontal view at 3 years of age, 1 year before injury, and then at 8 years of age, just before surgery. **B,** Frontal views before and 6 months after reconstruction.

Continued

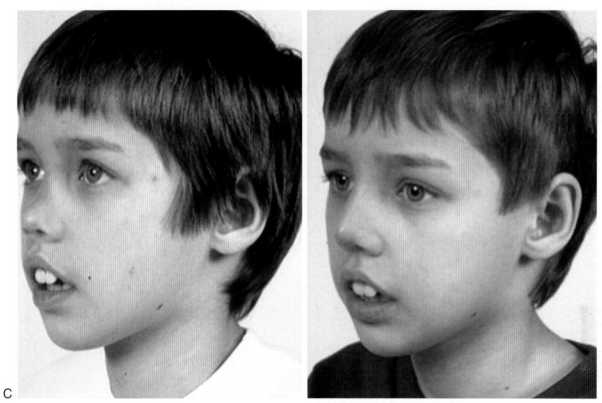

before & 6 months after nasal reconstruction

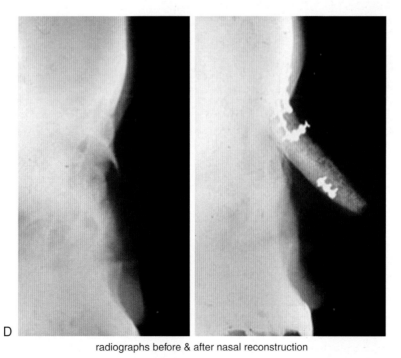

radiographs before & after nasal reconstruction

Figure 12.1, cont'd C, Oblique facial views before and 6 months after reconstruction. **D,** Lateral skull radiographs of the nose before and 6 months after reconstruction.

Continued

graft inset: naso-frontal process

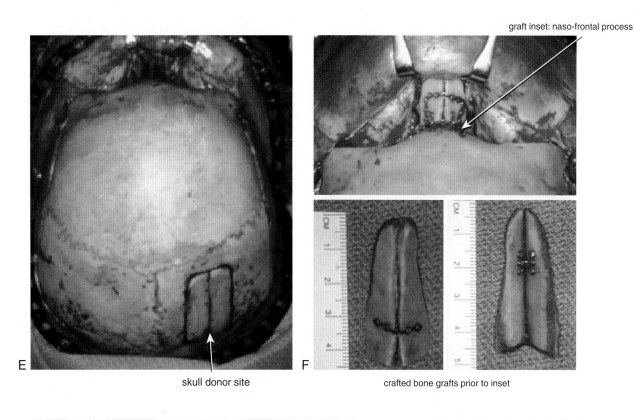

E

skull donor site

F

crafted bone grafts prior to inset

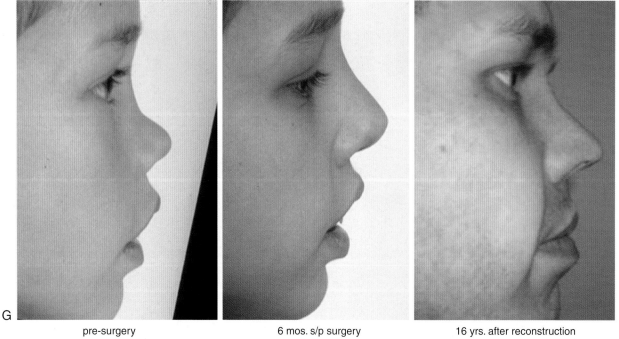

G

pre-surgery   6 mos. s/p surgery   16 yrs. after reconstruction

Figure 12.1, cont'd E, Intraoperative views through the scalp incision demonstrating the frontonasal region and the proposed right cranial vault donor site. **F,** Crafted full-thickness cranial bone grafts are shown before placement for nasal reconstruction. The close-up view of the frontonasal region shows the full-thickness cranial bone grafts fixated in place. **G,** Close-up lateral views of the nose just before surgery, at 6 months, and then 16 years after reconstruction. (A–G) From Posnick JC. Aesthetic alteration of the nose: Evaluation and surgery. *Orthognathic Surgery: Principles and Practice*, 2nd ed. (JC Posnick, ed., B Kinard, assoc. ed.). St. Louis: Elsevier. Ch. 38, Fig. 38-51, pp. 2076–2078; 2022.

References

1. Roe JO. The correction of angular deformities of the nose by a subcutaneous operation. *Med Rec.* 1891;40:57.
2. Weir RF. On restoring sunken noses without scarring the face. *N Y Med J.* 1892;56:443.
3. Israel J. Two new methods of rhinoplasty. *Arch Klin Chir.* 1896;53:255.
4. Joseph J. *Rhinoplasty and Facial Plastic Surgery.* 2nd ed. Leipzig: Curt Kabitzsch; 1931.
5. Posnick JC, Seagle MG, Armstrong D. Nasal reconstruction with full-thickness cranial bone grafts and rigid skeletal fixation through a coronal incision. *Plast Reconstr Surg.* 1990;86(5):894–902.
6. Millard DR, Mejia FA. Reconstruction of the nose damaged by cocaine. *Plast Reconstr Surg.* 2001;107:419.
7. Posnick JC. Aesthetic alteration of the nose: evaluation and surgery. In: Posnick JC, ed., Kinard B, assoc. ed. *Orthognathic Surgery: Principles and Practice.* 2nd ed. St. Louis: Elsevier; 2022. ch. 38.

13

Cosmetic Rhinoplasty

JEFFREY C. POSNICK, DMD, MD

Attempts to surgically alter the shape of the nose have been described for over 100 years. Cosmetic rhinoplasty was first reported to the medical literature in the United States by Dr. John Roe (1891) and in Europe by Dr. Jacques Joseph (1898).[1,2] The procedures were carried out under cocaine local anesthesia in the surgeon's office with the purpose to make a "smaller" nose that would be "less conspicuous" when viewed in a public setting. Dr. Roe recognized the potential hazards of carrying out a purely cosmetic facial procedure when he stated: "In all surgery about the face, it is necessary to avoid mutilation [when attempting to surgically correct the problem] since in many instances [the] operation [under consideration] might otherwise simply exchange an unsightly blemish for a [true] deformity."[1]

Dr. Joseph, as professor of surgery at the University of Berlin went on to publish the first comprehensive textbook covering the subject of cosmetic and reconstructive rhinoplasty in 1931.[3] Dr. Joseph described the rationale for completing his first cosmetic rhinoplasty. In the 1898 publication, he stated: "a 28-year-old landowner inquired whether I could make his nose smaller. He related that his nose was the source of considerable annoyance. Wherever he went, [people] stared at him, often he was the target of remarks or ridiculing gestures. On account of this he became melancholic [and] withdrew almost completely from social life. [He] had the earnest desire to be relieved from the deformity."[3] This fear of being judged negatively by others when seen in a public setting remains a common feeling by most, in all cultures, even in individuals with what might be considered a minor yet visible facial difference.[4]

Today cosmetic rhinoplasty has become a safe and relatively predictable procedure (see Figs. 13.1–13.4).[5-7] Individuals commonly request surgery to improve the shape of their nose but may not appreciate other facial dysmorphology that also affect their appearance, such as disproportion of the jaws (see Chapter 7).[8] Individuals requesting cosmetic rhinoplasty often also suffer from chronic obstructive breathing due to abnormal internal nasal anatomy. If so, they will benefit from simultaneous correction of the deviated portions of the nasal septum and reduction of enlarged inferior turbinates. For these reasons, successful rhinoplasty demands that the surgeon identify any baseline abnormal intranasal anatomy affecting breathing as well as appreciate the individual's overall facial dysmorphology affecting aesthetics before proceeding with a requested limited nasal cosmetic procedure (see Fig. 13.5).[8]

The surgeon's clarification of realistic facial aesthetic and nasal airway expectations prior to surgery and then executing a safe and predictable surgery is essential to achieving patient satisfaction. A cosmetic rhinoplasty procedure is typically carried out under general anesthesia on an outpatient basis, followed by discharge home to the care of a family member.

Letter from a Past Patient

Dear Dr. Posnick,

I am writing to let you know how happy I am with the results of my nose surgery. I feel so much more confident in the way I look. No one stares at me anymore! You have made me feel much more comfortable with myself every day which helps me at school and when with friends.

Sincerely,
Katie Williams

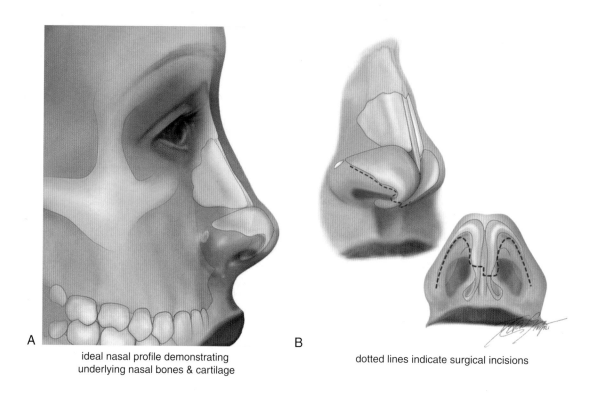

A, ideal nasal profile demonstrating
underlying nasal bones & cartilage

B, dotted lines indicate surgical incisions

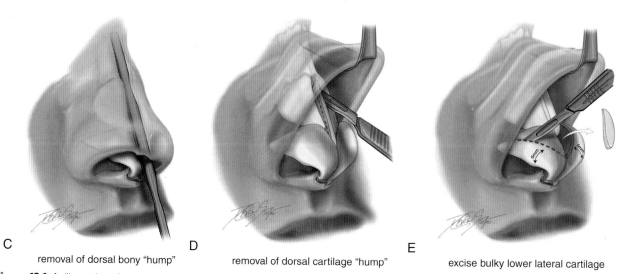

C, removal of dorsal bony "hump"

D, removal of dorsal cartilage "hump"

E, excise bulky lower lateral cartilage

• **Figure 13.1 A,** Illustration of optimal soft tissue and skeletal anatomy of the nose as seen in profile. **B,** Incisions that are used for an "open" technique rhinoplasty are demonstrated in dotted red lines. **C,** Removal of dorsal bony "hump" with a rasp. **D,** Removal of dorsal cartilage "hump" with a scalpel. **E,** Reduction of cephalic excess of lower lateral cartilages.

Continued

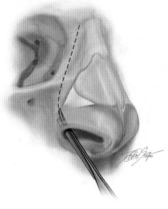

F

osteotome for nasal osteotomies

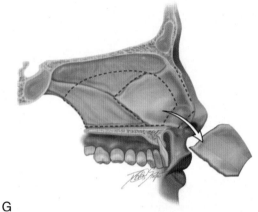

G

deviated nasal septum removed
cartilage graft for nasal tip

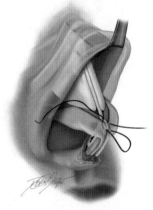

H

placement of septal cartilage graft
to improve nasal tip projection

Figure 13.1, cont'd **F,** Osteotome used to complete nasal osteotomy through intranasal incisions. **G,** Dotted lines indicate the extent of septum (bone and cartilage) removed to improve the airway. Inset illustration indicates removed septal cartilage that can be used as graft material to reconstruct the nose. **H,** Septal cartilage graft sutured in place. Lower lateral cartilages are sutured together and over the top of the graft to improve the appearance of the nasal tip. (A–H) From Posnick JC. Aesthetic alteration of the nose: Evaluation and surgery. *Orthognathic Surgery: Principles and Practice,* 2nd ed. (JC Posnick, ed., B Kinard, assoc. ed.). St. Louis: Elsevier. Ch. 38, Fig. 38-1, p. 1979, Fig. 38-8, p. 1994; 2022.

Figures continue

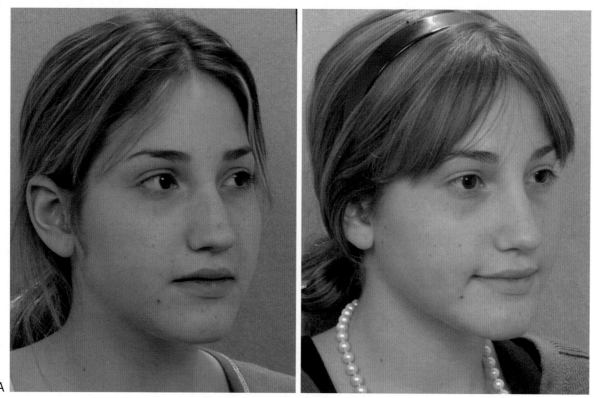

teenager before & after rhinoplasty

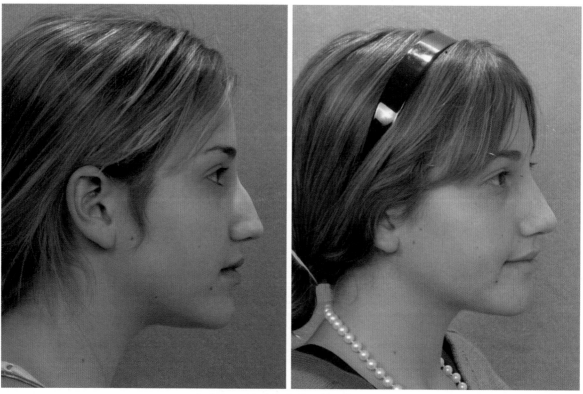

teenager before & after rhinoplasty

• **Figure 13.2** A teenage girl arrived with her parents and requested a reduction rhinoplasty. She also had difficulty breathing through the nose. She was otherwise with good facial proportions and therefore underwent an "open" rhinoplasty that included nasal osteotomies (in-fracture); dorsal reduction (bone and cartilage); nasal tip refinement (reshaping of the lower lateral cartilages [LLCs] and septal cartilage caudal strut grafting); septoplasty; and inferior turbinate reduction. **A,** Oblique facial views before and after surgery. **B,** Profile views before and after surgery. (A–B) From Posnick JC. Aesthetic alteration of the nose: Evaluation and surgery. *Orthognathic Surgery: Principles and Practice*, 2nd ed. (JC Posnick, ed., B Kinard, assoc. ed.). St. Louis: Elsevier. Ch. 38, Fig. 38-13, pp. 2003–2004; 2022.

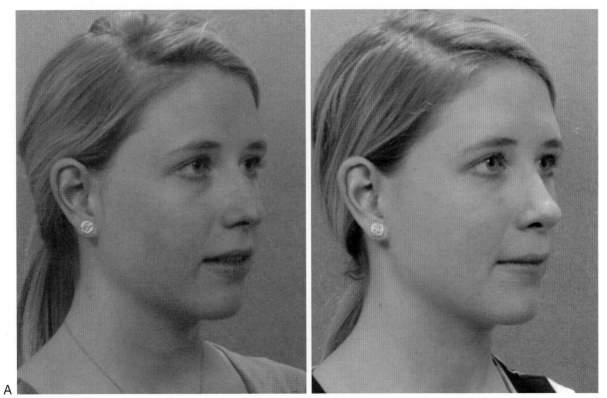

teenager before & after rhinoplasty

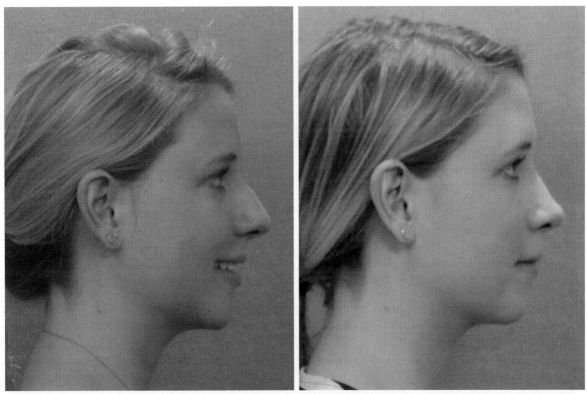

teenager before & after rhinoplasty

• **Figure 13.3** A teenage girl arrived with her parents and requested cosmetic rhinoplasty and the improvement of her nasal breathing. She was otherwise with good facial proportions and therefore underwent an "open" rhinoplasty that included nasal osteotomies (in-fracture); dorsal reduction (bone and cartilage); nasal tip refinement (reshaping of the LLCs and septal cartilage caudal strut grafting); septoplasty; and inferior turbinate reduction. **A,** Oblique facial views before and after surgery. **B,** Profile views before and after surgery. (A–B) From Posnick JC. Aesthetic alteration of the nose: Evaluation and surgery. *Orthognathic Surgery: Principles and Practice* , 2nd ed.(JC Posnick, ed., B Kinard, assoc. ed.). St. Louis: Elsevier. Ch. 38, Fig. 38-14, pp. 2005–2006; 2022.

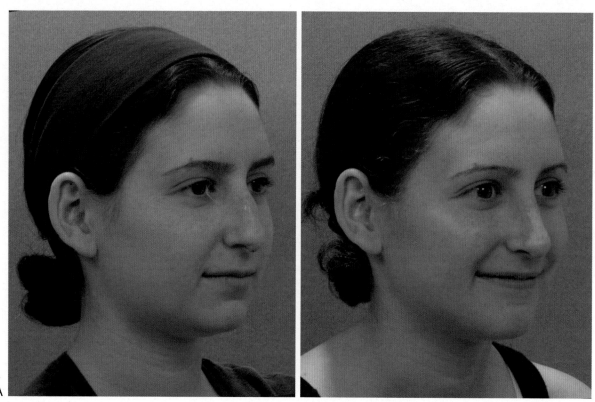

teenager before & after rhinoplasty & genioplasty

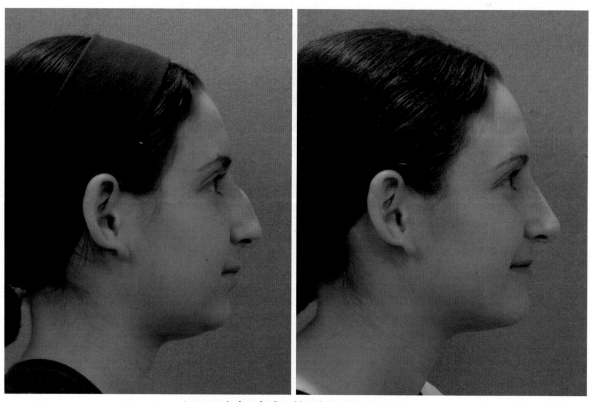

teenager before & after rhinoplasty & genioplasty

• **Figure 13.4** A teenage girl arrived with her parents and requested a "smaller and more attractive" nose. Rhinoplasty to reduce the dorsum and elevate the tip in combination with genioplasty to improve the profile was recommended. She underwent osseous genioplasty and an "open" rhinoplasty that included nasal osteotomies (in-fracture); dorsal reduction (bone and cartilage); nasal tip refinement (reshaping of the LLCs and septal cartilage caudal strut grafting); septoplasty; and inferior turbinate reduction. **A,** Oblique facial views before and after surgery. **B,** Profile views before and after surgery.

Continued

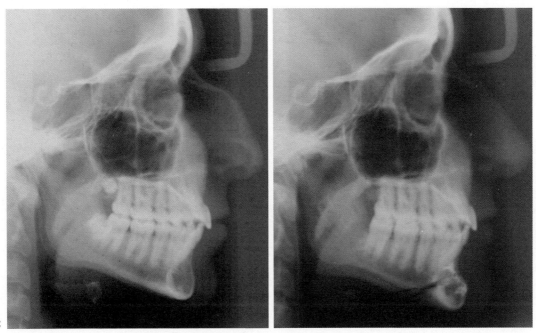

C

cephalometric radiographs before & after rhinoplasty & genioplasty

Figure 13.4, cont'd C, Lateral cephalometric radiographs before and after surgery. The extent of chin lengthening and advancement can be seen. (A–C) From Posnick JC. Aesthetic alteration of the nose: Evaluation and surgery. *Orthognathic Surgery: Principles and Practice*, 2nd ed. (JC Posnick, ed., B Kinard, assoc. ed.). St. Louis: Elsevier. Ch. 38, Fig. 38-15, pp. 2007–2008; 2022.

dorsal reduction (bone & cartilage) to remove "hump"

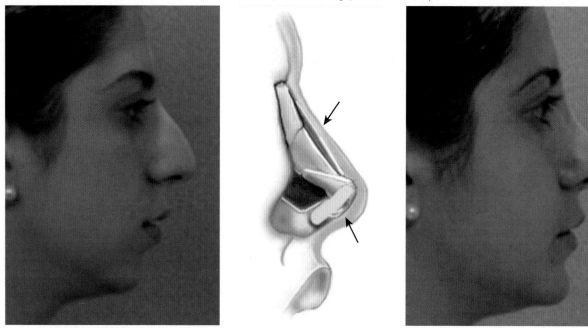

A

prior to surgery

cartilage graft to improve tip projection

s/p jaw reconstruction & rhinoplasty

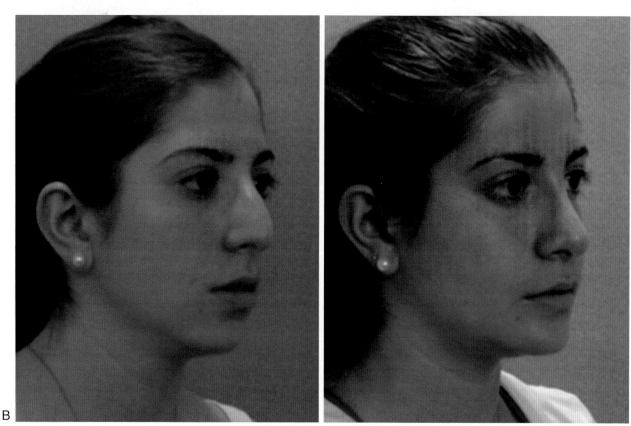

B

teenager before & after jaw surgery followed by rhinoplasty

• **Figure 13.5** A teenage girl arrived with her parents and requested a "smaller" nose. She was recognized to have a developmental dentofacial deformity as well as a nasal deformity. **A and B,** Close-up profile and full facial oblique views are shown before and after sequenced jaw reconstruction for a developmental dentofacial deformity and then, 6 months later after rhinoplasty. The rhinoplasty highlights the advantages of the combination of dorsal reduction (bone and cartilage) and nasal tip elevation (i.e., caudal strut [septal] cartilage grafting and lower lateral cartilage reshaping) as typically carried out to achieve objectives. (A–B) From Posnick JC. Aesthetic alteration of the nose: Evaluation and surgery. *Orthognathic Surgery: Principles and Practice*, 2nd ed. (JC Posnick, ed., B Kinard, assoc. ed.). St. Louis: Elsevier. Ch. 38, Fig. 38-23, pp. 2020–2023; 2022.

References

1. Roe JO. The correction of angular deformities of the nose by a subcutaneous operation. *Med Rec*. 1891;40:57.

2. Joseph J. Operative reduction of the size of a nose. *Berl Klin Wochenschr*. 1898;40:882.

3. Joseph J. *Rhinoplasty and Facial Plastic Surgery*. Leipzig: Curt Kabitzsch Press; 1931.

4. Newell R, Marks I. Phobic nature of social difficulty in facially disfigured people. *Br J Psychiatry*. 2000;176(2):177–181.

5. Millard DR. *Principalization of Plastic Surgery*. Boston/Toronto: Little, Brown and Company; 1986.

6. Sheen JH. *Aesthetic Rhinoplasty*. 2nd ed. St. Louis: Mosby YearBook; 1987.

7. Gunter JP. The merits of the open approach in rhinoplasty. *Plast Reconstr Surg*. 1997;99:863–867.

8. Posnick JC. Aesthetic alteration of the nose: evaluation and surgery. In: Posnick JC, ed., Kinard B, assoc. ed. *Orthognathic Surgery: Principles and Practice*. 2nd ed. St. Louis: Elsevier; 2022. ch. 38.

Appendix A

Future Directions in the Field of Facial Reconstruction

JEFFREY C. POSNICK, DMD, MD

Future directions in the evaluation and treatment of pediatric facial deformities will take advantage of new technologies. Cutting-edge innovations will include advances in: telemedicine; diagnostic imagery; biomaterials; prosthetic devices; surgical planning; operating room design; pharmacology; molecular genetics; advances in health care data collection; and use of artificial intelligence (AI). A spectrum of virtual and augmented realities will also change the way surgical training and planning take place and will democratize the availability of care worldwide.

Telemedicine: Telemedicine improves access for patient consultation and care. As our understanding of facial deformities improves, the transmission of up-to-date information and expert advice will become more readily available to both patients and surgeons worldwide. Telemedicine can even allow a distant experienced surgeon to literally walk the less experienced surgeon through a complex operation in real time.

Improved diagnostic imagery: Innovative computed tomography (CT) and magnetic resonance imaging (MRI) scanning technologies and image processing with improved accuracy will define the extent of skeletal and soft tissue deficiencies in children with malformations and deformity. The advanced imaging will more accurately define and locate the boundaries of tumors. The design of "fast" MRIs and "flash" CT scanning technologies will reduce and may even eliminate radiation to children altogether.

New biomaterials: Reliable biologic bone and cartilage substitutes used to replace missing parts or to augment deficient tissue structures within the craniofacial region will be readily available. This will avoid the need to either harvest the patient's own tissue or the need to use less favorable artificial materials that are prone to infection or rejection. These new materials will be available as pastes for the surgeon to free form the missing part or as prefabricated 3-D printed patient-specific skeletal units to accurately replace or to augment the deficient structure.

Improved prosthetic devices: The need to replace complex structures within the head and neck, such as missing teeth, jaw joints, components of the ears, the nose, and eyes, will remain with us. Innovative technologies and biomaterials will continue to improve the quality and success of dental implants, cochlear implants, custom temporomandibular joints, external ears, the nose, eye, and eyelid replacements to restore both head and neck function and facial aesthetics.

Virtual surgical planning: For the management of complex facial deformities in children, innovative software will use CT scan and MRI imaging data to virtually clarify absent or deficient skeletal components and determine optimal reconstruction. The seamless transfer of this information for use by the surgeon in the operating room will improve outcomes. The construction of accurate, user friendly, cost-effective cutting guides, jigs, and patient-specific fixation plates will be used to position and secure osteotomy segments in optimal locations at operation. These innovations will exponentially broaden the worldwide network of surgeons capable of performing complex facial reconstructive procedures for the correction of malformations. By first performing the operation in the "virtual" or "augmented" world (i.e., mock surgery dress rehearsal), either on a 3-D printed model or when wearing 3-D goggles that simulate the operative field, the surgeon will anticipate challenges, improve efficiency, and minimize errors.

Operating rooms of the future: Computerized responsive lighting in the surgical field will auto-adjust the intensity and direction to minimize glare and eliminate shadows for the surgeon. Fluid evacuation systems that instantly recycle suctioned blood safely will stretch the limits of surgery. Real time navigation systems will routinely be used to indirectly locate tumor boundaries, identify fractures, and optimize fracture reductions. Robotic-assisted surgery will improve visualization of deformities without collateral damage and also accurately dissect and separate tumors from the normal tissue planes. The surgeon's ability to safely distinguish the normal from the pathologic structures without need for direct vision will minimize complications and errors.

Pharmaceuticals: The development of new medications with limited side effects to prevent infection, limit swelling, relieve nerve injury pain, arrest degenerative bone and joint diseases (i.e., temporomandibular joint conditions). They will also play a role in shrinking and suspending the growth of congenital tumors (i.e., vascular malformations, fibrous dysplasia), and prevent, limit or reverse soft tissue scarring (i.e., due to trauma or surgical injury). This will improve the way that craniofacial deformities and head and neck tumors are managed in the future.

Molecular genetics: Innovative genetic testing to identify cleft and craniofacial malformations will be available. The ability to modify genes and even prevent mutations altogether through targeted medications (e.g., folic acid for neural tube defects) will have a dramatic impact on the occurrence of facial malformations.

Democratizing facial reconstruction: Two barriers to equitable access for comprehensive cleft and craniofacial patient care include lack of geographically available clinical expertise and finance. Enhanced funding at the federal and state levels for the care of children with facial deformities and dental rehabilitation needs will dramatically reduce hardship for families and communities. Both virtual and " hands on" simulation-based training will be essential components of surgical education in the years to come. Accessible simulated training will help to level the playing field for surgeons throughout the world. In doing so, it will improve access to safe and effective reconstructive surgery for children with complex facial deformities.

Accurate health care data: A child with a complex facial deformity may have undergone a variety of treatments and procedures at different institutions over many years. Each child's medical data needs to be integrated and readily available to avoid errors in future care. The use of a virtual medical assistant to maintain and update an individual's record continually and seamlessly from the womb to the present will be possible. Development of an accurate computerized nationwide registry to track the prevalence of pediatric facial deformities and the reconstructive procedures carried out will encourage the study of results and complications to improve future outcomes.

Artificial intelligence: We may live to see the transformation of artificial intelligence (AI) from having the ability to simply code hard data to a more human-like approach. AI will have the flexibility to process facts and ideas in an adaptive way and then analyze information from a variety of perspectives. In the future, AI may routinely clarify the comprehensive diagnosis of children with facial deformity and then recommend optimal treatment. Advice may include suggestions about the preferred timing, sequencing, and design of the reconstruction.

Appendix B

Final Thoughts

JEFFREY C. POSNICK, DMD, MD

Through an understanding of where we have come from and with the knowledge of what we can offer our patients today, the next generation of craniofacial and maxillofacial surgeons will no doubt carry the torch further down the road. It is from experience that I can say it is a path with false turns and deep potholes. The road wanders, and may even double back, but seen from a distance, it always leads in the right direction.

Never underestimate the difference that one person can make when they are single-minded, committed, persistent, and in it for the long haul. In the medical field, always search for the truth without accepting dogma at face value. Be an individual in your way of thinking. Have the will to be the odd man out. See an unmet challenge, develop a plan, and give it your all with one mind and one heart. Never lose your curiosity; have determination, maintain high standards, and use your special skills to do good work for others. Remember that there is no greater religion than human service. I have learned this from my mentors and have personally tried to follow in the same spirit.

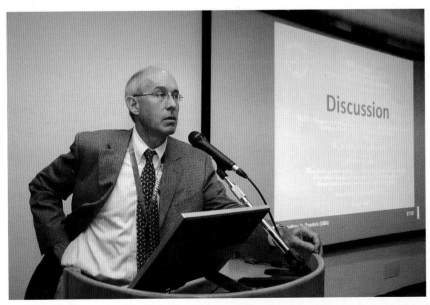

• Session during a surgical symposium in 2016. It's always great fun to share knowledge about advances in the field.

Practicing with a Reverence for the Past

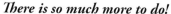

A central aspect of most pediatric facial deformities is the need for jaw reconstruction and dental rehabilitation. Optimal treatment typically requires thoughtful and experienced collaborative efforts from specialists in the fields of medicine, surgery, and dentistry. Today, our ability to successfully reconstruct an adolescent's jaw deformity is due to the pioneer surgeons and orthodontists that came before us. It is my belief that practicing surgery with a reverence for the past provides perspective and humility. Although there have been contributors from many in both disciplines, three surgeons and three orthodontists deserve special mention for their milestone contributions. These *surgeons* are Hugo Obwegeser, William Bell, and Hans Luhr and the *orthodontists* are Edward Angle, William Proffit, and Lawrence Andrews.

Obwegeser described a safe and practical way to section and reposition the maxilla (i.e., Le Fort I osteotomy), the mandible (i.e., sagittal ramus osteotomies), and the chin (i.e., intraoral oblique osteotomy). *Bell* utilized an experimental model to prove the biologic safety of orthognathic osteotomies. *Luhr* developed and demonstrated the use of small metal plates and screws for the practical and safe rigid fixation of all the bones of the craniomaxillofacial skeleton.

Concerning the orthodontist pioneers, *Angle* was the first to articulate the difference between a dental malocclusion and a dentofacial deformity and visualize the possibilities through elective jaw osteotomies. He challenged surgeons to consider osteotomies for jaw reconstruction. It was *Proffit* who recognized the need for a routine, collaborative, surgeon–orthodontist interaction to correct dentofacial deformities and the importance of assessing long-term outcomes. *Andrews'* major contributions are twofold: first, in recognizing the physiologic importance of using orthodontic mechanics to center the dental roots solidly in dentoalveolar bone; and secondly, to unapologetically recommend jaw osteotomies to achieve optimal facial harmony.

There is so much more to do!

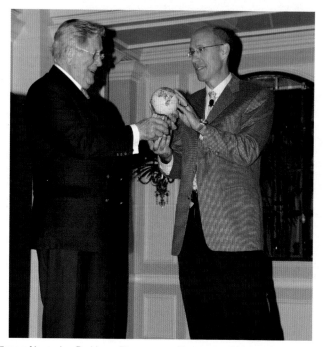

• In 2009, I had the privilege of honoring Dr. Hugo Obwegeser with an award for his pioneer contributions to the field of maxillofacial surgery.

Index

Note: Page numbers followed by "f" indicate figures "t" indicate tables and "b" indicate boxes.